LIMERICK CITY LIBRARY

Phone: 407510
Website:
www.lim____ ___ie/library
E____ ___ ___kcity.ie

The Granary,
Michael Street,
Limerick.

____ and b____ ____ued subjec' to 'he Rules of 'hi

Overcoming Common Problems Series

Selected titles

A full list of titles is available from Sheldon Press,
36 Causton Street, London SW1P 4ST and on our website at
www.sheldonpress.co.uk

The Assertiveness Handbook
Mary Hartley

Breaking Free
Carolyn Ainscough and Kay Toon

Cataract: What You Need to Know
Mark Watts

Cider Vinegar
Margaret Hills

Coping Successfully with Period Problems
Mary-Claire Mason

Coping Successfully with Ulcerative Colitis
Peter Cartwright

Coping Successfully with Your Irritable Bowel
Rosemary Nicol

Coping with Anxiety and Depression
Shirley Trickett

Coping with Blushing
Professor Robert Edelmann

Coping with Bowel Cancer
Dr Tom Smith

Coping with Brain Injury
Maggie Rich

Coping with Chemotherapy
Dr Terry Priestman

Coping with Dyspraxia
Jill Eckersley

Coping with Gout
Christine Craggs-Hinton

Coping with Heartburn and Reflux
Dr Tom Smith

Coping with Macular Degeneration
Dr Patricia Gilbert

Coping with Polycystic Ovary Syndrome
Christine Craggs-Hinton

Coping with Postnatal Depression
Sandra L. Wheatley

Coping with a Stressed Nervous System
Dr Kenneth Hambly and Alice Muir

Depressive Illness
Dr Tim Cantopher

Eating Disorders and Body Image
Christine Craggs-Hinton

Free Your Life from Fear
Jenny Hare

Help Your Child Get Fit Not Fat
Jan Hurst and Sue Hubberstey

Helping Children Cope with Anxiety
Jill Eckersley

How to Beat Pain
Christine Craggs-Hinton

How to Cope with Difficult People
Alan Houel and Christian Godefroy

How to Keep Cholesterol in Check
Dr Robert Povey

Living with Asperger Syndrome
Dr Joan Gomez

Living with Autism
Fiona Marshall

Living with Fibromyalgia
Christine Craggs-Hinton

Living with Food Intolerance
Alex Gazzola

Living with Loss and Grief
Julia Tugendhat

Living with Lupus
Philippa Pigache

Living with Rheumatoid Arthritis
Philippa Pigache

Living with Sjögren's Syndrome
Sue Dyson

Losing a Child
Linda Hurcombe

Making Relationships Work
Alison Waines

Overcoming Loneliness and Making Friends
Márianna Csóti

Treating Arthritis – The Drug-Free Way
Margaret Hills

Understanding Obsessions and Compulsions
Dr Frank Tallis

Overcoming Common Problems

Coping with Pet Loss

Robin Grey

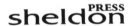

First published in Great Britain in 2006
Sheldon Press
36 Causton Street
London SW1P 4ST

The author and publisher have made every effort to ensure that the external website
and email addresses included in this book are correct and up to date at the time of
going to press. The author and publisher are not responsible for the content, quality
or continuing accessibility of the sites.

All names and details contained in the case studies are
fictional but are based on typical bereavement situations.

British Library Cataloguing-in-Publication Data
A catalogue for this book is available from the British Library

ISBN-13: 978–0–85969–962–4
ISBN-10: 0–85969–962–5

1 3 5 7 9 10 8 6 4 2

Typeset by Deltatype Limited, Birkenhead, Merseyside
Printed in Great Britain by
Ashford Colour Press

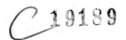

In memory of my Aunt Rene and Bwino

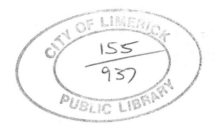

Contents

	Introduction	1
1	The human/animal bond	5
2	Deciding when it is right to end a pet's life	13
3	The impact on you	24
4	Pet loss and children	42
5	Missing: when a pet is lost	61
6	Accepting loss and grief	66
7	Pet loss in later years	71
8	Losing a service dog	78
9	Remembering a pet	82
10	Deciding about another pet	87
	Conclusion	94
	Useful addresses	95
	References	101
	Further reading	102
	Index	103

Acknowledgements

Thanks to the following: Maggie Beresford, Jo Ann Dono, Clare Guest, Colin Heard, Phil Woods, and everyone who was so helpful in giving insight from their personal and professional experiences.

I also wish to thank my partner Terry, Theresa, Mum and Dad for all their encouragement and support during the writing of this book.

Finally, thanks to Fiona Marshall, Sally Green, Steve Gove and everyone at Sheldon Press.

Introduction

Losing a pet can be extremely stressful, and the average life span of a pet means that we may potentially experience many such losses in our own lifetime. Each loss will be different and will depend on the unique relationship that has developed through the years during which the pet was with us. Such loss not only represents the end of a special relationship, but can remind us of religious and cultural traditions from which we may have become distant. However, among those who either have not experienced it or who seem indifferent to its impact, there remains a great deal of misunderstanding of what the loss of a pet can mean.

Pet loss sometimes happens at times when we feel that we can cope and have the resilience to accept it. Yet there are also times when we feel less able to cope. Such losses can be sudden or unexpected. The loss of a pet, whether from illness, accident, theft, abandonment or old age, can happen when we ourselves are going through a time of vulnerability or transition. It is then that the loss becomes harder to manage.

Supporting someone through the loss of a pet requires time, empathy and understanding. These qualities are sometimes in short supply; many people do not understand the bond that can form between humans and animals and encourage others to 'get over it' before they are ready to do so. This book is intended for everyone who has been directly or indirectly affected by pet loss, whether through personal experience or through knowing and supporting someone who is grieving for their pet.

When children lose pets, they are often facing their first experience of loss and are going through what can feel like a major bereavement. Helping them learn through this experience, validating their loss and involving them in letting go can be invaluable. It is reassuring for children to have the support of adults who recognize their upset feelings while enabling them to gain some perspective on what has happened.

Similarly, for the increasing number of people who live on their own, pets may have become a kind of substitute family, requiring care and attention and communicating a childlike dependency. Following a difficult period in your life, or a period of significant change, it sometimes feels that pets offer an emotional security that is not available elsewhere. Your choice of pet may reflect this need: some pets are naturally independent while others require more looking after, and taking the responsibilities of pet ownership seriously can enable us to satisfy a need within ourselves.

Whether we are alone or not, throughout our lives pets give unconditional acceptance in a way that may be hard to find in other relationships. Our pets can be the holders of our secrets, witnessing the emotions that we do not want others to see.

As humans, our experience of loss can be profound and can touch us in ways that we do not expect. We may need time to mourn. It may feel that we will never recover. The loss of a loved pet can seem like one of the hardest losses. There is hope, though. By examining ourselves and our own reaction it is possible to see that this often unpredictable loss can draw us closer to others who have shared the same experience. Losses can make us feel vulnerable and misunderstood. At such times it is useful to seek out the experience of others in order to validate our own experience and to gain support.

The human/animal bond is timeless. It is defined by history, cultural traditions and family ties, and by our need to feel attached. The loss of a pet can feel like the end of an era in your life. Grieving owners feel that they will never recover from the loss of their companion. Yet we do recover and eventually move on.

Of course, death is inevitable. As living beings we are all mortal and at risk of terminal illnesses. It may feel difficult to accept this when mourning our pets, especially if we feel that they died too young or were victims of an unexpected accident. The emotions and thoughts attached to such losses are intense. It can feel as if we are mourning the loss of a part of ourselves. With the awareness of mortality, however, comes an opportunity to celebrate the gifts of life that are given to us in our relationships and attachments with others.

You may be reading this book following your first experience of pet loss, or you may be anticipating a loss. You may want to help someone who is currently grieving. It can be difficult to know how to respond if you are supporting someone following such a loss – your approach may be welcome, or it may be seen as an interference in what feels like personal grief.

Some people feel relief following the loss of their pet, especially if the pet had been suffering. Others can be more matter-of-fact about it. The dilemma of how to respond can be hard to resolve.

Whatever your experience, this book aims to help you to answer some of these questions. It is vital to remember that the loss of our pets gives us an opportunity to show our love, to connect with aspects of ourselves and to find a sense of hope for the future.

The impact of pet loss can extend beyond owners themselves. There is evidence that vets too find it extremely stressful, and that, in some cases, it can form an emotional burden that is just too hard to bear. The suicide rate among vets is nearly four times the national average and double that of doctors or dentists, according to research published in the British Veterinary Association's (BVA) journal. The report states that women vets are particularly prone to depression and suicide, though one concern is that male vets may be hiding their emotions and not seeking help. Richard Halliwell, a former president of the Royal College of Veterinary Surgeons and one of the report's authors, suggests that the suicides could be related to the stress of putting down animals. Prof. Halliwell also spoke of the emotional stress caused to vets by having to care not just for the animals, but also for owners, who often treat their pet as they would a child.

I hope that this book may, therefore, help relieve some stress among vets as well as among pet owners.

1

The human/animal bond

'We do not die who live on in the hearts of those we have
loved'
— inscription from a pet cemetery gravestone,
Jesmond Vale, Newcastle upon Tyne

There are three points that need to be considered when looking at the
human/animal bond.

First, our relationship with pets is historically defined. We may
have become less dependent on animals financially in modern
societies, but they still play a crucial role in many urban and farming
communities. They fulfil an equally crucial role in giving status and
making us feel wanted and needed. Pets can help people to restore
their self-esteem, creating a sense of belonging. Having pets can
facilitate our instinctive qualities of caring and nurturing.

Animal behaviourists have studied the ways that humans interact
with pets. This has enabled them both to explain the connection
between pet and owner and also to appreciate the processes of
communication entailed, involving instinct and interaction. The
establishment of a link between ethology (the study of animal
behaviour) and human attachment was important in enabling scientists
in the mid-twentieth century to develop theories that have since been
used to help people understand parenting and psychological processes.

Second, the attachments that we develop and maintain with our
pets are thrown into focus when we experience pet loss. It is implicit
in the work of the psychoanalyst John Bowlby that the degree of loss
we experience is related to the strength of attachment that we hold to
the attached subject. Therefore, any unresolved or insecure attachment can result in a high degree of stress following a loss. Bowlby
cites examples of other species, such as geese, orang-utans and
chimpanzees, who engage in searching behaviours when confronted
with the loss of a loved object.

The child psychologist Boris Levinson made further specific
findings showing how children can benefit from regular contact with
pets. In his classic study, *Pets and Human Development* (1972), he
provides evidence for the previously theoretical link between pets
and humans.

5

This human/animal bond can be strengthened by the unconditional love shown to people by their pets. One owner commented that 'no matter what difficulties I faced during that time I knew that Missy was there for me . . . she wouldn't take sides . . . I knew she needed me and that made all the difference.'

Moreover, there are many stories about pets that come to rescue people in physical danger or alert those in distress. It was reported, for example, that Abraham Lincoln's dog had been howling and running around the White House just before his assassination. Pets act on instinct for survival and for protection. They anticipate danger from a distance and their senses are much more highly tuned than we sometimes acknowledge.

Lastly, many people hold the view that we are all part of life's creation, and this belief fosters a mutual dependency between us and animals. For religions including Hinduism, Islam, Christianity and Buddhism, respect for all living beings is a central tenet of their faith. These beliefs, as expressed through religions and philosophies throughout the world, have been well established for centuries. Their message reaffirms the importance of looking at 'all creation' as being interdependent for survival and mutual respect. You do not have to adhere to any particular religion to have a strong sense that what was special about your pet continues after it has passed on.

It can be useful to think about how pets, like humans, have a life cycle with defined stages. Just as we have our youth, middle years and old age, so do our pets. This helps us to identify with our pets and to recognize how their lives are evolving naturally as they move through life. Many animals, by showing signs of withdrawal and being quieter than usual, may demonstrate an innate awareness that they are coming to the end of their lives. This need not alarm you, but can prepare you for change.

The significance of attachments

In considering pet loss it is relevant to think about your early experience of having pets. This can help you to understand how and why you are feeling as you do, and the way your previous experiences have affected the way you look at loss now. The loss of a pet is not easy to deal with. It can trigger memories of previous losses and unresolved attachment issues. This may not cause you major difficulties. If it does, however, then after reading this book you might want to consider further help, detailed at the back of the book.

Pets, and dogs in particular, seem to understand attachment well. They need us as we need them. They depend on us, and their day's routine will be dictated by their need for walking and eating which we have to provide. At times when we feel down, we appreciate their company and they, in turn, offer companionship and unconditional love.

However, we may not have experienced a pet's dependence on us since childhood. Children can become attached to their pets as if they are special 'soul mates'. As adults, the forming of an attachment to a pet can be the start of a very special relationship that connects with part of us that may have been neglected or has not been nurtured. If so, then it will have added significance as it will be a bond that will feel special and unconditional.

The experience of 'separation anxiety' following the loss of a pet is recognized as a factor in the loss process. This anxiety follows as a direct consequence of the loss. Anyone who has nursed an ill pet will recognize the protective instinct that emerges at such times. If your pet was euthanized or put to sleep it is common to experience anxiety when you are left alone without it. The dependency that comes from being in close proximity to a pet, followed by the empty space that is left afterwards, can make the anxiety of separation – at least in the short term – harder to bear.

Factors that strengthen human/animal bonds

A number of important factors have been cited by pet owners in explaining the origins of their attachment to their pets. Here are a few:

- Their pets were crucial in helping them through a difficult time in their lives.
- Early attachments to pets began in childhood and this set a pattern.
- In childhood, a special bond developed between them and a pet which has helped them through a difficult emotional period of change or transition.
- Pets are a link to previous losses they have experienced, such as bereavement and separation.

- They have had to rescue their pets from a near-fatal accident or attack.
- A lot of time and money has been invested in providing their pet's healthcare and happiness.
- They have given their pets human characteristics. This may indicate a special closeness, but may indicate an over-identification with their pets. (The term 'anthropomorphism' describes the giving of human characteristics to pets.)

The above list is by no means exhaustive, but does indicate the varied – and perfectly valid – reasons for the attachments that develop between pets and owners. The strength of the bonds that exist between pets and their owners helps to explain how, as a society, we are seen as being pet lovers. Pets provide unique, unconditional love to people in a way that often cannot be put into words.

Therapeutic value of the human/animal bond

The value of owning a pet, or of having access to pets in our everyday lives, is widely recognized. Studies on the subject show that having a pet can benefit families' communication and common purpose, can lessen conflict between people and add to the compassion that they have for other living things.[1]

It is also claimed that having a pet can help to reduce stress by lowering blood pressure levels. A study in Australia showed that men who owned pets had significantly lower systolic blood pressure than those without pets.[2] Pets have also been identified as being a source of psychological and therapeutic support for survivors of childhood sexual abuse; when recounting their stories many survivors have told of the comfort that they found in the special relationship with their pets.

The therapeutic value of touch is also important. As a society we are still often inhibited in showing physical affection to each other, which is often permitted to take place only in certain socially sanctioned environments. This may explain why touching and showing affection to pets is more visible and accepted in society.

However, the loss and grief felt for pets that have died or whose lives have had to be ended is still something usually experienced in private. Just like other forms of bereavement, it is typically hidden from view, as we often feel embarrassed or inhibited in expressing grief.

It may be useful at this stage to consider some points relating to your attachment to your pet or the pet you have lost. You may feel that the focus of your relationship with your pet was in the strong attachment that you had from an early stage of their time with you. Or you may feel that it was the close physical nature of your relationship with your pet that signified the closeness that you have had. The loss of touching and being touched by your pet can be felt particularly keenly by recently bereaved owners. One owner summed this up when she stated:

> A few months after Patsy died I was sitting in the chair. I thought I had been coping without her quite well, but it was only when I put my hand down to the side of the chair to give her a stroke that I remembered that she wasn't there. I had got so used to her being by the side of me during the evening that it came as a bit of a shock to realize that she wasn't there any more. I did that several times afterwards too. It made me think that our bond was really quite strong, though I never thought about it much when she was with me.

The bond established by touch is based in the very early experiences of life. Touch continues to make us feel connected to the world around us. It makes us feel secure and part of life. And as we get older, it assumes a greater importance as there may be fewer opportunities for unconditional touch, hugs and love.

Pets as psychological protection

Having a pet can nurture the care-giving part in us which is a fundamental aspect of our psychological health. In many psychiatric histories taken following the onset of illness, losing a pet has often been cited as a contributory factor in a patient's subsequent breakdown. Psychiatrists will take note in bereavement histories of pet losses, as they are deemed to be significant to the bereaved owner and can be a significant factor when considering depression and breakdown.

Patients often attribute part of their distress to the loss of a pet. Conversely, pet ownership can be viewed as protecting against ongoing distress. It has also been found in the noting of psychological histories that children's cruelty to pets or small animals can be indicative of psychological disturbance. Pets, in effect, offer us psychological protection and their loss can make us more vulnerable.

No matter what pets you have – from horses to fish – in terms of coping with your pet loss it is the strength of the bond that will dictate and determine the extent of your grief.

Accepting when the bond will be broken

Inevitably, as pets get older or become ill there are warning signs that the special bond that you have sustained through the past years will eventually be (physically at least) broken as they approach the end of their lives. It can be hard to accept this and it is understandable to want to deny it. Preparing for bereavement of any kind can be exceptionally difficult. We push it to the back of our mind, despite the fact that common sense tells us that no living being is immortal.

Small signs of decline or ill-health can make us feel panicky, and we may rush to negative conclusions when faced with a pet whose health is obviously deteriorating. If you have past experience of the situation you will probably find this easier to accept, although it may bring back unpleasant memories from when this happened with previous pets.

It is important to notice any changes that take place with your pet, such as different eating habits. Older cats, for example, can become fussy in what they eat as their senses of taste and smell change. It is advisable to keep a record of what and how much your pet eats, especially if it seems to have become less interested in food. Taking this information to the vet can be helpful in enabling him or her to look into possible causes of the changes.

All vets will know, judging by your pet's age, what old age or 'geriatric' problems to look for. Being aware of what can develop enables the vet to catch such problems early, before they become too pronounced.

Depending on your previous experience and your relationship with your pet, you may either be anticipating bad news or be shocked by what you have heard. When bad news is confirmed it can take some time to sink in. The mere possibility of a serious illness, whether through old age or not, can be hard to accept.

It is likely that in anticipating the loss of your pet as it approaches the end of its life, there will be some ambivalence about your feelings. You don't want to lose your pet but you don't want it to suffer needlessly. You recognize that no life goes on for ever but you would like some more time together. You can see changes in your pet but you don't want to acknowledge them. You want the bond to remain intact, yet you are having to accept that it will have to change.

Town and country

Whether you live in a rural community or an inner city, your immediate environment will affect how you live with your pet and also how you will approach its loss. In rural and farming areas there can be a greater variety of animals. The loss of a pet may be felt more acutely when pets are surrounded by a rural context that values pets as part of a lifestyle that is not accessible in the city. The relationship between people and horses, one which is predominantly rooted in the countryside, demonstrates clearly the nature of the human/animal bond.

Losing a horse or pony

The relationship between people and horses is one that can start from a very early age. The non-verbal communication that can typify this relationship is built on mutual respect. Bonding with a horse can be a very intimate process that can take months, if not years, to establish, and there is always the risk that a horse may reject you. One owner commented:

I viewed the relationship that I had with my horse as essentially a psychological one. He knew that I was in control yet there was respect between us ... I was very aware that this relationship could flip over to a position where he was in control ...

Bonding with a horse can require a huge amount of investment. Consequently, the death of a horse can be a traumatic experience, especially as the bond that has been established has to be so carefully nurtured.

Losing a horse through sudden injury can of course be very difficult. The choice of administering a lethal injection or shooting the horse is not one that is easily taken. To maintain the dignity of an animal that is in intense pain, however, it can be the kindest course of action to save it from further suffering.

It is a measure of the intensity of the emotional bond that some owners of horses will choose not to be present when a horse's life is ended. One owner said:

> I knew that he was going to be shot that morning but I couldn't be there. I knew that my best course of action was to do something completely different that morning . . . I tried to act as if nothing had changed, but I was deeply affected by it for weeks afterwards. I knew that it was right to end his life but I realized how attached I had become . . .

One of the strengths of being a part of a community that values horses and ponies is that such communities are very supportive. If you face the death of a much loved animal then all those working at the stables will be understanding and will rally round to offer support. Traditionally, such communities accept the inevitability of death through illness or accident, and this can be helpful at such times.

Conclusion

When considering the loss of an animal that is close to us, it is important to recognize the bond that exists between pet and owner. This bond can be very strong, and can be the source of the grief that we experience on the death of a loved animal. Many of our personal reactions and feelings can be involved with this bond that draws us close to an often unexpressed sense of attachment. It can be hard to acknowledge that such a bond exists until we face loss and separation from the pets close to us. More often than not, we are faced with making decisions that dictate our pets' lives, and this potentially leaves us with feelings of guilt and responsibility. These issues are explored in the next chapter.

2

Deciding when it is right to end a pet's life

It is exceptionally hard to have to make the decision about when to end a pet's life, something which often has to be done following a vet's diagnosis and advice. Many people describe it as being one of the most difficult decisions that they will ever have to make. You may question whether you made the right decision, even though you know that it was in the best interests of your pet to prevent it from suffering. This is completely understandable and highlights the responsibility that comes with being a pet owner.

In addition, you will undoubtedly be feeling sad and stressed. Whether or not the news was expected, a degree of adjustment to the new situation that you face is still required. We often yearn to ignore what has just been said and hope that it will go away. Unfortunately, to deny the truth that is facing us makes decision-making even more difficult.

Of course, in an ideal world all of our pets would gradually get older and die naturally. This is what we hope for: that we can let life take its course so that our pets are spared any illness or suffering. If your pet died in its sleep due to old age you will have a different experience of pet bereavement. Nevertheless, even though you may have been expecting this to happen some day, and despite the knowledge that no living being lasts for ever, the experience of loss is still sudden. It may seem to be a blessing to you that you were spared having to make the decision to end your pet's life. However, it is often reported that unexpected death leaves us feeling shocked, having had no prior preparation or idea that it would happen. The subject of natural death will be covered later in this chapter.

Some people find themselves becoming pragmatic when faced with the difficult option of euthanasia; they know in themselves that they face choices and are clear about what they think and what they feel is in the best interests of their pet. However, when you are feeling vulnerable yourself it is also common to feel doubt about making such a decision.

Discomfort about having the power, as humans, to decide if and when to end an animal's life can weigh heavily on some people. It can make the situation that we face more difficult and leave us with feelings of guilt and indecision.

Anticipating loss

Whatever your circumstances, when a pet approaches the end of its life or is given a terminal diagnosis there is the reality of impending loss. This sense of loss can be overwhelming, especially when it is unexpected. It is common to experience a degree of shock when the news that you may have been dreading is made known. Grieving begins at this point, and justifiably so.

As your pet moves through the different stages of its life you may have noticed many variations in its activity levels and inquisitiveness. On the other hand, you may have given little attention to minor variations in behaviour and noticed only significant changes. When it becomes apparent that time is catching up with our pets, it can feel as if there is not enough of it left.

It is easy to wish to block out the advancing years of our pets and the reality that the time remaining to them may be short. But we all recognize that reality, even if we do not wish to see it. If you are concerned about the changes that you have noticed in your pet, do talk to someone about it, as this will ease the anxiety. By sharing your worries you are not only giving voice to them but having them validated by someone you trust. If it is subsequently necessary to contact the vet, then you will be more prepared for change.

Euthanasia

The option of euthanasia will not be one you take lightly. The term euthanasia itself means 'a good death' (from the Greek *eu* meaning 'good' and *thanatos* meaning 'death'). It is the hope of all pet owners that the end of their pet's life will be peaceful and can be achieved without remorse. However, achieving a peaceful transition for yourself following the loss of a pet can be more difficult, as feelings of guilt and anger may remain. Bearing in mind that it may have been the kindest course to end your pet's life can help to alleviate some of the initial guilt that you may experience. Reasons why euthanasia may be considered the best option can include:

- Your pet may be in physical or mental pain which is increasingly

obvious to you by its demeanour and behaviour. You may also
have noticed a change in its behaviour towards you.

- The condition of your pet, as diagnosed by your vet, is long term
  and causing your pet distress, or appears to be getting worse.
- Your vet is no longer able to limit the suffering of your pet. This
  can be the deciding factor for many owners, as they do not wish to
  cause their pet further distress by needlessly prolonging its life.

These reasons appear to be clear, and when you think about them it
may seem that they are obvious. However, when faced with the
reality of making this decision they may seem less straightforward.
But you will no doubt want to do the best you can; it can help to
write down the reasons why euthanasia is being advised.

Tackling indecision

Indecision can feel like muddled thinking. Ideas and doubts go round
in circles with no apparent resolution. You feel as if you are caught
up in a dilemma that cannot be resolved. Are you the sort of person
who makes decisions on your own, or do you feel more comfortable
taking advice? Is your distress preventing you from making a
decision? The following advice may help:

- Try to step back from your situation and allow yourself time to
  think.
- If you make the decision on your own, remember times when
  trusting your own judgement has served you well before.
- If you find it helpful to talk to other people you trust, allow them
  to hear your fears.
- Indecision does not have to stop you from coping. Try to set a
  realistic point where you can stop thinking and then make a
  decision. Satisfy yourself with knowing that you allocated time
  for reflection which helped you make that decision.

'I feel like I am playing God'

Our discomfort at having to make the ultimate decision about ending
another being's life can go to the heart of our own beliefs and
principles. You may have wished for your pet to have a natural
death, but the reality you face is different. Focusing on the reality of
the situation can help you to determine what is in the best interest of
your pet and, in time, this can be consoling.

Even with the advances made in veterinary sciences, there are limitations to what can be done to prolong a pet's life. However, it can be comforting to know that although, ultimately, the sources and origins of illness may be out of our control, we do have a choice about whether to act on the interventions that are available to alleviate suffering.

Of course these are personal, ethical and moral issues that you have to come to in your own way and your own time. Consulting your vet and finding someone to talk to about your concerns can be helpful when facing fears or reservations.

Helping you make the decision

Making decisions that are literally about life and death can be extremely difficult, especially when considering the unique bond that you have with your beloved pet. The following suggestions may be helpful when approaching this difficult task:

- Talk to people who know you and your situation. This will enable them to stand by you as you make the decision.
- Think about what is right for your pet. This may require you to separate your pet's needs from your own.
- Think about other people who have been in the same situation. Talk to someone who has had a similar experience to yours and ask what helped them. You may, in turn, be in the position of helping someone else one day, and your experience will be valuable.
- Think about the positive responsibility of being a pet owner rather than the negative consequences of having to make the difficult decision. This should help you to feel less burdened by the necessity of making the decision and enable you to make it in a clearer way.
- There is no one right moment to end a pet's life. It will become apparent, however, if your pet is in pain or is suffering. More often than not, this becomes the guide for such a decision. Your wish for your pet to be spared suffering can become evidence that you did the right thing.

It can be a mistake to make decisions when you are distressed by potential loss. You are likely to want some time to think in order to make the right decision. Have a chat with your vet about the prognosis and the likely outcome before you reach a decision. The decision has to be yours and has to be done in the best interests of your pet. You may also be able to sense whether your pet is experiencing pain and suffering.

Letting a pet go can also afford it dignity. Death is inevitable for every living being. Your responsibility as a pet owner affords you the unique opportunity to look after, care for, and guide a pet through life and death. When the time comes for you to let your pet go, whether through natural or assisted death, you are witness that it has been given the protection and love that is necessary and desirable.

Using your experience

In deciding when to let your pet go, it is likely that the first time will be the most difficult. You may feel that lack of experience holds you back from making what you feel is a clear decision. Get help from the expert, your vet. Visits to the vet are essential to monitor your pet's health and provide an opportunity for you to ask questions about your pet's general condition.

There are many books available that can advise on the behavioural and physical indications that accompany changes in the health of pets as they age. If you have faced this process before it should be easier to cope with, but remember that each pet will be different and will react differently. With experience you will learn how you yourself react and be sure when the time is right to let your pet go.

How you can help someone else

Supporting a friend or relative who is faced with the loss of a pet, either through euthanasia or from natural causes, can demand a degree of tact. How you do this will depend on how well you know the person concerned. However, you can provide vital support to the person you care about when they are experiencing a period of loss and readjustment.

If you are supporting someone who faces the end of a pet's life, it can be hard to know how to respond. You may feel regretful about the loss and sad on their behalf, but also slightly detached from it. It can be hard to empathize if you have not shared their experience. The following points are worth bearing in mind:

- Avoid pushing them into decisions that you think would be right for them or that would suit your own agenda.
- After the loss of a pet, people can feel isolated in their grief. Help by being available but avoid 'taking over'.
- Avoid suggesting a replacement pet soon after the loss. Any such decision should be made by the person concerned, and they may resent such a suggestion at this point in a desire to assert their own control over a particularly difficult situation.
- As well as support, people need space following a loss. Experiencing a loss can, in the short term, make you feel unable to assert control, as if matters are out of your hands. Be sensitive to this, and try not to 'take over'.

Self-doubt

It is human nature to feel a sense of responsibility when we have been invested with power over another living being. Because of the strong bond that existed between you and your pet, it is inevitable that you will be left asking 'Did I do the right thing?' This can often follow in the weeks and months after euthanasia, when the sense of loss is strongest and you have time to reflect on that loss.

A number of owners have described how, following the euthanasia of their pet, their self-doubt left them wondering 'What kind of person am I?' Self-doubt takes away our sense of perspective. It can be pervasive and may allow feelings of guilt to linger. It can make us question our own ability to do what is right. One owner recalled:

> When I was advised by the vet to have her put down I still didn't know if I was doing the right thing. Usually I am able to make decisions at work ... I manage seven staff and have to make decisions quickly, but this was different. I felt for a few days that I didn't know myself.

When we are caught up in grief it can seem hard to see things objectively. Many people have described how, following the loss of their pets, they were left with a void or empty space that became filled with mourning and worry. This can temporarily take hold as we readjust to the new situation without our pet.

There is no need to carry this burden alone. Sharing your doubts with someone you trust can be helpful in gaining reassurance that you made the right decision. Reading this book may also enable you to begin to let go of your doubt. We make decisions, however hard, based on the information that we have at the time, the prognosis given to our pets and following a period of knowing that our pets are coming to the end of their lives.

It is important to remember that self-doubt is part of the grief process. Your feeling of responsibility stems from being a good pet owner. This is the key to helping you to start moving from doubt to having a more positive perspective. The complex questions involved in being a care taker – having to act on behalf of your pet with love and care – mean that it can sometimes take time to develop a perspective on your loss.

Did I make the right decision?

In retrospect it occasionally feels that the wrong decision has been made. This can feel terrible at the time, but is likely to be a reaction to your immediate distress. It is easy to look back once it is too late. That is why it is so important that you take time to make the decision and consult those you trust – your vet, family members or friends who can comfort you and, if necessary, remind you of why you made the decision.

No one wishes to inflict unnecessary prolonged suffering on a dearly loved pet. There are times, though, where you may feel unable to make the right decision and rely on others to guide you with their care and knowledge. The feelings of guilt and anger that often result from a loss or bereavement can be strengthened by our own sense of responsibility. Letting a pet go can be an act of love and care, but it can trigger feelings of anger and guilt. (These are discussed in the next chapter.)

Sometimes it feels that the right decision – such as the desire to prolong a pet's life – was made for the owner but the wrong decision for the pet. This may only become apparent in retrospect. The following case study shows the common experience of many who face this dilemma.

Case study: Sally

Sally knew that there was something wrong with Lucky, her cat. Lucky had been showing signs of distress for the past couple of weeks and had been crying a lot. She was having trouble walking, had lost weight and appetite, and Sally feared the worst. She made an appointment with her vet and, after initial examination, the vet advised an exploratory operation. This was set for one week's time and Sally was asked to bring Lucky back then.

During that time Sally was very upset indeed. She spent time crying on her own and spending lots more time with Lucky. She felt it was important for her to do this because she thought that the time remaining might be short; it was important to value the time they had even if everything was going to be OK. Instinctively, though, she felt that something was wrong and went back to the vet for Lucky's appointment with a sense of dread.

Sadly, the exploratory operation revealed that Lucky had inoperable cancer. Sally faced the options of taking her home or asking the vet to end her life. The vet and staff were extremely supportive, but no one could tell Sally what to do. In the end, she took Lucky home because she wanted to spend just a little more time with her. It was clear after another ten days, though, that Lucky was getting no better and was beginning to experience more distress. Sally took her back to the vet's and she was euthanized.

In the following weeks, Sally was understandably upset by the whole experience. The past few days had been distressing for her and she began to doubt if she had done the right thing in bringing Lucky home when she was inevitably going to lose her. The next couple of months were difficult and Sally felt guilty that she had prolonged Lucky's life for her own benefit.

In time, Sally recovered from the loss, but the experience of shock at the news and her instinctive reaction to take Lucky home for some extra time was not easy to deal with. She recognized Lucky's suffering and now felt guilty at prolonging her pet's life. Yet she could not have known how long Lucky had to live and comforted herself that, when Lucky became visibly distressed, she had saved her from further suffering. She also recognized in herself that it was the desire to pretend nothing was wrong that had led her to want to take Lucky home. The following days had allowed her to say her goodbyes and accept the new but sad situation.

The role of a pet owner or guardian is not an easy one and is fraught with moral and ethical dilemmas. As humans, we can feel the discomfort of being able to advocate for pets, while also holding the power to end their lives in a way that is often not legally possible for ending human life. Sometimes you will not know what you think about the decision to end a pet's life until it confronts you head on.

Situations like this can complicate mourning and lead to protracted or extended grief. If you have faced this type of situation, it may be helpful to consider the following:

- Remember the reason that you made the decision to have your pet's life ended. It is easy to let feelings of guilt or subsequent indecision make you feel bad.
- You will not have made the decision without the advice of the vet and taking into account the likely prognosis. No one can be absolutely sure how long a pet will survive, but you will have thought about the vet's advice and so will not have acted alone.
- The desire to prolong life is a common reaction when faced with death of any kind. In pet death it is easy to use it as a bargaining tool, as there is the possibility of setting the time for a certain end to the life.
- By making the decision when there is a clear terminal diagnosis, you are preventing further suffering. It is important that your vet explains the prognosis clearly so that you are left with few doubts after the end of your pet's life. It is helpful to view your vet as an ally who has supported the decision that you have made.

When a pet dies naturally

It is understandable to wish for your pet to die from natural causes, or without assistance. It is the hope that your pet will reach the end of its life without suffering or pain. Your pet's life cycle has been seen through to its ultimate conclusion without distressing either it or you. You may have made a decision some time ago that you would only engage the vet in ending your pet's life if there was no other way to keep its dignity.

A natural death can bring with it the hope of a period of acceptance from us, and a gradual letting go that we can at least anticipate if not control. It may be a comfort to know that your pet died at home in familiar surroundings. Yet the actual loss, and the reaction to it, can be the same as if you had to make the decision to end your pet's life. The stages of loss still have to be worked through, although they may not be quite so intense as when the death is sudden or unexpected.

If your pet dies naturally, you may believe that its loss is somehow in the right order of things. But grief will still follow, and it can never be predicted how this will affect us. However, we can never prevent death and it can help in coping to reflect on the fact that you did the best you could to ease the way for your pet.

The role of pet crematoria

Increasingly, owners are choosing to have their pets cremated following death. Cremation is seen as the best solution for a range of practical and environmental reasons.

As cremation can happen very soon after a pet's life has ended, it is understandable that it may be a sad and often distressing time for owners. However, it remains a dignified way to mark the end of a pet's life. Pet crematoria can be found across the country and they offer a number of different cremation services. The best crematoria offer individual or private cremation, providing owners with a safe and private setting in which to say goodbye.

A spokesperson for Cambridge Pet Crematorium agreed that it is important for vets or veterinary nurses to offer choice when an animal dies at the practice – either through euthanasia or natural causes – and to recognize pet owners' different needs when they require cremation for their pet:

> It is important to acknowledge the grief of people who have very recently lost their pet. By explaining the options available to them we aim to give them choice. Individual service and support is extremely important when they face their loss, especially if it has been sudden and unexpected. Many people are shocked and unprepared by their grief. We encourage people to think about what they would like in advance and plan their pet's cremation, so that they can concentrate on their grief when the time comes. It's a bit like making your own will and specifying the type of funeral you would like because that makes coping easier for the family.

If you wish to have your pet cremated and do not know the kind of questions to ask, the following points may help you:

- Ask about individual cremation. This is where your pet is cremated on its own. Following the cremation you can receive your pet's ashes back in a casket or urn. You can decide after the cremation what you would like to do with the ashes, such as interment or scattering. This service can be of comfort, enabling you to know that the remains you receive are those of your pet. This is important, as a pet is often seen as a family member or companion. Its death is a significant loss that deserves to be given dignity and afforded respect. It is important to ask for individual cremation if this is what you require.

- Attending the cremation can play a significant part in acknowledging the loss. You may feel that being witness to your pet's journey helps you to make the loss more real. Religious and cultural beliefs can be marked in ceremonies that take place in the 'farewell room' kept aside for the purposes of owners who wish to make a spiritual, religious or personal farewell to their pets. Crematoria do recognize how losing a pet can impact on our sense of life and its meaning.
- If you decide not to attend the cremation but ask to have your pet's ashes returned to you, then this can also help to signify the finality of your loss. It is then your choice what you do with the ashes. Ask about this, so that you know you will receive the ashes.
- Many crematoria have gardens of remembrance where you can have a memorial or plaque with a special inscription in memory of your pet. You can also choose to inter or scatter your deceased pet's ashes here. Gardens of remembrance are designed to be places of peace and tranquillity that reflect the special bond and spiritual nature of pets and the gifts that they bring to people's lives.
- Experienced advisers are available at the best pet crematoria to assist people who need to talk through their loss. Asking about this service will give you more information or further contacts.
- If there has been uncertainty about the reasons for a pet's death, it is possible to request a post-mortem examination from your vet. Understanding why the pet died may help you achieve closure. Pet crematoria will be familiar with such circumstances and will offer assistance and information, as well as presenting the pet in the best possible way for viewing following what can be a distressing procedure for the owner.
- Staff who work at pet crematoria are invariably trained and experienced in pet bereavement and the effect that pet loss has on owners. If you require someone to talk to while you are arranging your pet's cremation, you can expect an empathic and understanding approach from them.

Contact details for pet crematoria are listed at the back of the book.

3

The impact on you

Your decision to have a pet in your home will have changed your life. It may have been carefully thought out over a long period or arrived at more spontaneously. Much thought has gone into deciding what pet to have, choosing the right breed and making sure it is compatible with the rest of your household. However the decision was made, from the moment you get a pet and bring it into your home a bond will be established between you.

As the years pass, that bond will have grown stronger as you have cared for and looked after your pet. Whether you have had the pet since it was very young or taken in an animal that needs special care, this bond, and your subsequent dependency on each other, will make any anticipated or actual loss hard to accept.

It is not only after an animal's passing that we experience loss. The process of loss begins from the moment you notice a difference in your pet's responsiveness, a change in its movement or behaviour – and if this is pronounced, then expert help will be needed. The warning signs may start to show themselves when you notice that your once lively dog is not running to the door or jumping up to greet you as he used to. A cat that was once independent and spent hours exploring now prefers to curl up and sleep in your lap. As your pet slows down, its activity levels decrease and age and illness begin to take their toll.

It is now that you truly begin to realize that your pet is not going to live for ever. You will have known this for a long time. However, seeing an animal's physical and mental decline will make thinking about the end unavoidable.

Myths about pet loss

Following the death of a pet it is common for others to hold preconceived ideas about how you will react. If this is your first experience of losing a pet, then it can be hard to reconcile the way you imagined things to be with how they actually turned out. Myths, or even stories passed to others by experience, can sometimes give a false impression of what lies ahead. Here are a few of the common myths or assumptions made about pet loss:

- **'Everyone will be sympathetic to you.'** Your loss may be taken seriously by some people who either understand what it is like to have a significant loss or who have lost pets themselves. However, not everyone has unlimited sympathy. Some people may make light of or trivialize your loss, causing hurt and further distress to you as you try to cope with what is already a stressful experience.
- **'It won't take you long to recover from pet loss.'** Recovery depends on many factors, including your experience of past losses, the circumstances of losing your pet, your relationship with your pet and the situation you find yourself in now. Trying to minimize a loss can be counterproductive and sometimes causes further reaction later. It is important to give yourself time to recover. It doesn't always take a long time but it can take longer than you think.
- **'Getting another pet will replace the one you have lost.'** It is common to think that having a pet – any pet – to replace the one you have lost will guarantee your getting over pet loss. It can often help but will not, of course, replace the unique relationship that you had with your lost pet. Concerned relatives and friends of people who have lost pets sometimes rush in too quickly either to talk about or actually physically replace a pet for a grieving owner.
- **'Children get over these things quickly.'** It may take a long time for a child who has built up a strong relationship with a pet to acknowledge its loss. It depends on the nature of the relationship and the age at which the loss occurs, but it is wrong to assume that all children will react the same way. The loss of a pet is one of the first experiences of loss that a child is likely to have. The child needs time to make sense of it and so the expectation that they will be less affected is not true. The importance of helping children cope with the loss of a pet will be explored in detail in the next chapter.
- **'Older people will get over it quicker as they have more experience.'** It is sometimes assumed (especially by those who do not have pets) that the loss of a pet will affect older people less. Losing a pet can cause loneliness, magnifying feelings of isolation, and can be very difficult to cope with. The loss of a pet may mean the loss of companionship. It doesn't matter how many times people have experienced such a loss, it doesn't make it any easier – especially if it coincides with other losses or with a period of change in your life. The impact of pet loss on older people will be explored in Chapter 7.

- **'Losing a pet gets easier if you have one or two pets already.'** Pet owners often say that each of their pets has its own definite character and that they have a completely different relationship with each pet. Your family (including pets as members) will still be bereft following the loss of one pet, while behavioural changes often occur in the other pets, who have, after all, themselves experienced a loss.
- **'Your life will get back to normal soon enough.'** This may be true for some people but not for others. Losing a pet has been said by some people to be like losing their only friend, or even like losing a child. The relationships that we forge with our pets can be life-changing because of the strong bond that is established. After the pet's passing it may take a long time for a feeling of normality to return. Even when you have recovered from your loss, it will have made a change in your life, something that is important to remember.

It has to be recognized that the loss of a pet happens on two different levels. First, there is the actual loss of the pet you have loved and known for years. Second, and perhaps more difficult to work through, is what having a pet represents to you. Many people say that having a pet is like an extension of themselves. A pet can represent a precious sense of freedom that you feel you have lost. It can represent a desire to care for another being, or may be seen as holding a sense of spirituality that we can identify with in some way.

Stages of loss

Loss does not happen all at once. It is a process that takes time, from the recognition and acceptance that your pet is unwell through to the end of its life. Depending on the circumstances, healing and recovery from this loss can be long and hard. When thinking about how we manage loss, it is helpful to see it as being a process that can be worked through in different stages.

Not everyone experiences all these stages. Nor do they come in a neat, predictable order. If only the response to loss was like that, so that there was a tidy end to what is often an unpredictable time. It can be hard to control the response to loss in the early stages, especially if you feel overwhelmed by what has happened. Fear and grief do eventually pass, though, and the experience of loss can give way to a greater meaning. The rest of this chapter outlines the main stages of loss that lead to eventual acceptance.

Shock

It is probable that you will experience a degree of shock if you have been told bad news about your pet. This particularly happens if you have had no warning. However, even if you knew at the back of your mind that your pet might be terminally ill, to have this confirmed may feel devastating. A shock reaction may also follow a traumatic event, for example if your pet is involved in a road accident.

Our initial emotional reaction following any sudden death is characteristically a feeling of numbness. This often occurs as the news begins to sink in, and can also manifest itself as a physical sensation. The other physical reactions most commonly associated with shock are feeling faint, nausea, shaking, feeling 'frozen' or feelings of dissociation, as if you are temporarily not involved with what is happening around you. Shock can necessitate medical help, so do not hesitate to access this if necessary.

Denial

Denial is an instinctive response to the shock of a loss, and is commonly experienced as a physical or psychological numbness to feeling. Denial could be described as our instinct to block out what has just happened. It can sometimes be manifested by continuing as normal, as if a loss had not actually happened. It can sometimes feel as if it is a kind of forgetting that anything has changed. One dog owner said when talking about her experience:

> For a few days after the accident I had convinced myself that nothing had changed and I carried on as normal. I even told someone new at work that I had two dogs when in fact I had only the one now. Part of me refused to accept that the accident had happened. I think it made it difficult for people at work to talk about it with me for a couple of weeks, because I was so convinced that nothing had happened.

Another owner's experience followed a rally in her pet's health:

> I just didn't believe that she was so close to death, because the day before she died she seemed better than she had for months. She seemed to be much more alert and I hoped, somehow, that I

was going to have some extra time with her. It was like I had her back again. I couldn't believe it when she finally died, as I was sure she was turning the corner the day before.

A common manifestation of denial in pet loss is the belief, on hearing news from your vet, that there has been a mistake in diagnosis. Disbelief is our way of fending off the knowledge that something bad has happened. 'There must be a mistake' or 'They must have another pet's results' are common reactions to dealing with bad news. We hope above all else that there has been a mix-up, and we may ask for a second opinion that may or may not be available.

Of course, denial has a function. It stops people having to face the awful reality of the loss that they have just experienced or the news that they have just heard. It allows them to delay, however briefly, facing grief and the separation that follows. For people supporting someone who is in denial about the loss of a pet, especially if they are now left on their own, this stage is hard to cope with. The symptoms of acknowledging the loss may be put back indefinitely while denial continues.

If you have experienced this you will know that it does not last, but is a way of blocking out emotional pain which can tide us over until the worst of the shock subsides. It can be damaging if it continues too long and prevents change. Delayed grief or lack of grief can cause problems.

However, grief cannot be 'made' to happen. We all respond differently to loss, and what might seem an appropriate reaction in one person may not be for another. We cannot assume that because someone isn't grieving for their pet, they are in denial and surely must start grieving soon. The closeness of the relationship is a good indicator of the expected grief reaction. Routines that were centred on your pet can be hard to alter, and the negotiation of these can indicate the degree to which you are adapting to life without the pet.

If the death of a pet follows the comparatively recent loss of a significant person in your life, then this can be another reason for denial. To have to face the loss of a beloved pet that directly reminded you of someone you loved and who also loved that pet can seem too hard to bear. The association a pet may have with the past and with times that are now gone can make your current loss unbearable and push you into denying that it has happened.

If this has happened to you, it may feel that you are both denying that the pet has died and finding it hard to accept that the loved person has gone as well. It can often bring back grief that you thought you had worked through, so that you think more of the person you have lost. It can feel like a double loss, or it may feel that another part of your loved one has gone – a part that was keeping their memory alive.

In contrast, there might also be some relief that the person did not have to experience the loss of their pet, and died knowing that you would care for them. Your care for their pet was a continuing part of your love for them and it is hard when that continuity ends. You may want to approach this loss differently, as a kind of final chapter that will eventually bring a sense of completion to your longer-term grief.

Bargaining

When a pet is ill and has only a short time to live, we typically wish that we could do something to make it better. This translates into saying things such as 'If they could prolong his life I would promise to take more time to be with him.'

In a sense this is an extension of denying that the inevitable is going to happen. We hope with a much loved pet that something – anything – can be done to keep it with us for a little longer. Of course, this invariably leads to disappointment and the bargaining fails. It can also be found in the relationship that pet owners have with their vets when faced with a pet in obvious pain; the wish to keep the pet with us for longer can become a wish for its suffering to end.

One of the main functions of bargaining is to keep some hope alive. The possibility of a cure, of a different dietary programme, of doing something that may keep our pet healthier for a little longer is a common feature of trying to hold back ill-health and eventual loss. If you are supporting someone who is facing loss and is in the bargaining phase, it is important to recognize that hope is part of their eventual acceptance. To be confronted with too much truth about the inevitable too early on can be unnecessary and may interfere with the loss process. One pet owner summed this up well:

I was trying to reconcile my wish to keep him with my wish to let him go in peace. My vet helped me to see that the illness he had was affecting his quality of life so much that letting him go was the best thing to do. I spent so much time hoping for a positive outcome – that he would get better or that the cancer would somehow disappear. But I had so much weighing up to do in my mind between keeping him and letting him go. In the end letting him go was best for both of us, but it was hard to see it at the time.

Of course, bargaining inevitably has to give way to the eventual acceptance of your pet's illness. However, its importance comes in defending us at times when we need to know that there is still hope. It can also reveal the depths of our frailties and so give us a period of time to assimilate what we expect will be the outcome when faced with bad news.

A common temptation when faced with the loss of a loved pet is to replace it with another one as soon as possible. Deciding to get another pet is, of course, a personal decision. It can be seen as a compromise. Care must be taken to avoid replacing your pet in the hope that you will thereby avoid all the grief of losing your previous pet, as the result could be that you displace or fail to acknowledge the necessary loss that you feel. Deciding whether or not to get another pet will be covered further in Chapter 10.

Searching

Following a loss it is common to search for what we have lost. Even though we know that our pet is no longer with us, it can take a while to get used to the idea. We react by searching for our pet, or for another one that is reminiscent of what our pet was like. Seeing another pet that looks or acts like ours can disconcert us for a split second. We may think for a moment that our pet has come back, until we realize that it is actually no longer with us. This can remind us of the reality of our loss.

It has been said that searching is similar to denial, in that it is hard for us to accept when a loved one has gone. It is easier to search for our pet or identify aspects of it in others, and for that brief moment we can think that our pet is back again. Do not worry about this, as it is a common reaction to having experienced a recent loss.

Anxiety

Another stage that can affect people following a loss is anxiety. Having recently been witness in some way to the loss of a pet can be an upsetting experience and can make us worry more, almost instinctively. Any such loss can be a shock to our psychological system and it can take time to get used to the new situation without our pet.

Anxiety following the loss of a pet typically focuses on whether we made the right decisions when the pet was alive, while feelings of anxiety can also accompany being alone. We worry about what might happen next or what might befall our other pets. The experience of losing a pet can trigger worry about those who are close to us and make us reflect on things we hold dear.

If you find that you are experiencing significantly greater worry or anxiety following your loss, contact your GP. In addition there are a range of self-help techniques that many people find helpful, such as yoga, relaxation techniques, including deep breathing or listening to calming music, and talking therapies. Contact numbers and addresses are listed at the back of this book.

Anger

When facing loss it is common to experience feelings of anger In his book *Bereavement*, Colin Murray Parkes identifies anger as occurring fairly early on in the grieving process. It should also be viewed as a normal part of that process. Many people still think that anger is a negative emotion, particularly following a loss. In fact it is a perfectly normal reaction to a situation that can often feel out of our control. It is what we do with our anger that is important.

Anger is an understandable and normal reaction to any loss or bereavement. Before jumping to conclusions about who, if anyone, is to blame it is helpful to reflect on where your anger lies and how it is directed. Our feelings of impotence, unfairness and helplessness when faced with the loss of a pet can be powerful and should not be underestimated.

Anger can feel very potent. It can have a strong impact on our well-being. Managed well, it can make us feel strong and in control, yet if badly handled and turned in on ourselves it can lead to stress, raised blood pressure and depression. It can also lead us to blame others rather than face our own acute emotional pain following a loss. As pets are dependent on us for their health, well-being and care, when this cannot be sustained – for whatever reason – we may be left feeling helpless and unable to do anything. In pet loss there are often complicating factors which can contribute to a sense of loss and, at times, of injustice.

As a pet owner, being angry on behalf of your pet when faced with loss may well feel justified, but it is harder to manage. Your anger may be directed at the vet who you believe to be responsible by not doing everything they could to save the pet. Even if you know that they did their best, blaming them can seem to be a justified response.

Anger towards the vet

Despite the fact that vets clearly explain the reasons for having to euthanize pets, it is not uncommon for pet owners to feel angry towards their vet following a loss, particularly if there has been some doubt about the pet's prognosis.

Listening to bad news is different from actually hearing it. It can take some time to accept the implications of the news you have just heard. If your pet still seems quite alert although a terminal diagnosis has been made, or if you feel that it still has some good days, then this can lead you to want to blame the person who gave the diagnosis. Your vet should involve you in explaining the reasons for his or her advice, but ultimately it is your decision about when to end your pet's life.

It is important to remember that your vet is only the carrier of the bad news, and is not personally responsible for your loss. Remember that vets are working within the limits of their profession and are accountable for their ethical standards like other professions. If you are dissatisfied with the care your pet received, then making a complaint can help. However, it is important to think about whether you are doing this more through unresolved grief than a justified grievance over lack of care.

The relationship that you have with your vet is another key factor. Try to maintain a good relationship with your vet and practice so that you feel that they are supporting you. Building up a sense of trust over the visits will help to reassure you of your vet's professionalism.

Most of all, it is important to be clear about the reasons for your pet's illness, the prognosis and the reasons the vet gave for having your pet euthanized. If you are clear about the reasons then this should make it easier for you to accept the loss. If you remain unclear, then ask again to have the reasons explained. There should be no embarrassment about asking for reassurance about the reason, and it could save you a lot of heartache.

Anger towards yourself

In the absence of having anyone else to blame, directing anger towards yourself is a common reaction. This is usually experienced as guilt, which is covered in the next section. It is easy to blame

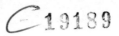

oneself when there is no obvious person or institution to be angry with. If you had someone else to blame then it might make it easier. Invariably, though, following pet loss there is a degree of self-blame and anger that is directed inwards.

It is important to recognize when you feel angry with yourself, as it can prevent you turning in on yourself further. You may have been left feeling that you didn't do enough for your pet and that you are in some way to blame for its death. Coping with this feeling on your own can be very hard and can make you feel that you are letting it get the better of you. Expressing your anger can be very therapeutic and can help you avoid stress.

There are a number of self-help measures that can assist you to manage anger. Sometimes it is hard to completely let go of the guilt that we impose on ourselves, but it is possible to manage it more effectively:

- Talk to other people about it. This can enable you to develop a sense of perspective. It is likely that you are blaming yourself, rather than that others are holding you responsible.
- Think about ways that you can change how you view your current relationships with pets. Despite doing all you could for your pet in the circumstances, you may be feeling that you did not do enough. It is easy to focus on what you think you should have done better; instead, try to think about your positive qualities as a pet owner.
- You may have unreasonable expectations about what you can do for a pet that is ill. Try to think about what you feel is good enough, rather than imposing on yourself unachievable expectations for the level of care that you provide.

Anger towards God or a higher being

The loss of a dearly loved pet can result for many people in anger towards God. The death of a pet can make us question the meaning of all life and cause a crisis in faith or in long-held beliefs. Rather than blaming a vet or themselves, it is understandable that some people blame a higher being.

As we question losses and bereavements we often are searching for answers. Some people suffer a crisis of faith when someone or something precious is taken from them. However, given time this can lead to a resolution, and the questioning can be positive. Whatever your beliefs, such anger is usually temporary.

It is common for people to say that a loss makes them feel they are at some kind of 'crossroads'. This can be interpreted in different ways, but it suggests the existence of several options that are not clear at present. It may feel that choices will come from this fork in the road, whether about beliefs or decisions. Above all, it is important to allow yourself time, following any loss, to work out what you really want.

You may even feel anger towards the pet that died. 'How could she leave me?' 'Why did he have to die so young before he had lived a full life?' Again, this is an understandable reflection of the dependency that you and your pet have on each other. You may feel bad about being angry with your pet after it has died, but do remember that this is all part of the loss and grief reaction that is felt by many.

Anger towards those responsible for the death of a pet

Anger is particularly hard to manage if your pet has been killed by the intended or unintended actions of others. It is understandable to feel acute and powerful anger towards those responsible for a pet's death if it was beyond your control. It is hard to overestimate the emotional impact of such losses, and they can lead to feelings of intense rage towards those responsible. Forgiveness may not be possible and it is important not to feel pressured to forgive.

When we fail to assuage our anger towards others for the loss of our pets, there is the risk that ultimately we will turn this blame on ourselves and search for a reason why we didn't do more ourselves. This can delay our eventual recovery.

Guilt

The loss of a pet is often accompanied by feelings of guilt or self-reproach. It is in the nature of our pets' dependency on us, and our responsibility to them, that the end of the relationship leaves us feeling helpless or that we did not do enough. You can be reassured by everyone around you that you acted in the right way, but that may not be enough. You still feel justified in holding on to the belief that you did the wrong thing.

Guilt is also related to the power between human and pet. We have the capacity to end an animal's life in its best interests or to witness its decline into the final stages of life. Invariably, though, we are faced with difficult choices at the end of a pet's life and often find that we are in a 'no-win' situation. Try to remember this when tackling your own feelings.

Guilt is often retrospective. It occurs when it feels too late to do anything. It leaves us feeling lost and helpless, angry and impotent. It seems easier to blame yourself than to accept that you acted within the limits of your knowledge and circumstances at the time.

It is common following a bereavement of any kind to experience a degree of 'survivor guilt'. We feel bad that we are still here when the pet or person we loved is not. This feeling may be less powerful when facing the loss of a pet than when a person close to us has died, but it is nevertheless one that is often expressed following a decision to end a pet's life. It can also follow the inevitable feeling of emptiness that comes after euthanasia.

Guilt can maximize grief at exactly the wrong time in the loss process. It can trigger negative thoughts that are hard to get rid of, and it is easy to go over and over the same thoughts and feelings because we haven't sorted them out. This can be debilitating for anyone who experiences it, and because we hold our guilt individually it is a very personal emotion to work through.

Guilt is unproductive. It can make us feel passive and as if we are to blame. It can also cover up strong feelings of anger. It stops our progress towards a resolution. It can make the grief process longer to resolve. The following factors are frequently given as contributing to guilt:

- Prolonging a pet's life too long. The desire to keep a loved pet with you for as long as possible can, in retrospect, lead to the feeling that you kept it with you for too long. Sometimes pets rally towards the end of their life, leading to false hope and accompanying guilt; we wonder at such moments whether they could have lived a little longer. Having to reach a decision when your feelings are in conflict with the ethical needs of your pet can amplify later doubts. Take advice and reassurance from those involved with the treatment of your pet.
- Being unable to pay for better treatment somewhere more specialized. We are all limited to a greater or lesser extent by money. In the wish to get the best possible treatment available for our pet, you are limited by what you can afford and what is available. No animal is immortal and we have to recognize the limitations of both what we can afford and what is medically possible. If you have explored all the practical options, then you have done the best you can.
- Not being with your pet at the end. For whatever reason, you may

have been prevented from being with your pet at the end of its life. Even if this was so, it did not stop you from loving, caring and wanting the best for your pet. People often go over the reasons why they could not be there at the end, and invariably it has to do with their being prevented by circumstances beyond their control.

- Failure to prevent accident or theft, or attack by other animals. While your instinct is to protect, most pets are naturally curious and independent. We cannot possibly watch over them every minute of the day, and accidents do sometimes occur. Coping with lost or stolen pets will be dealt with more fully in Chapter 5.

Resolving guilt

If you find yourself unable to resolve feelings of guilt or self-doubt following the loss of your pet, consider seeking help. Holding feelings of guilt over a long period can be destructive. It also has a powerful effect in allowing us to blame and feel bad about ourselves. In this way guilt can be extremely hard to put aside when we reflect on how we acted or did not act.

The dependency that pets have on us, especially when they are ill or suffering, can make it easier for guilt to take hold. It may help to talk to someone who can see things from a different perspective. Talking to someone independent can help you to let go of these feelings and to recognize that you did what you could at the time. Remembering the following points may help to resolve feelings of guilt:

- It is an intrinsic part of our responsibility towards pets and their dependency upon us that we often feel we cannot do enough.
- We have to make decisions that are in the best interests of the pet. Drawing on the experience and expertise of other people enables us to make informed choices.
- Talking about feelings of guilt is better than keeping them to yourself. In order to eventually recover from pet loss, it is important to work through any feelings of guilt.

Depression

Depression often follows loss and is a normal part of the grief process as we readjust to new situations. However, it is often accompanied by feelings of loneliness and helplessness in response to the new situation we face.

If you feel that your loss is not being taken seriously (as can unfortunately happen with pet loss), this can make things worse. Even if you told people before its death that your pet was ill, you may receive a polite but indifferent response to your loss that can make you feel that very few people understand.

Depression is common following a loss. It is often a manifestation of other feelings that are turned in on themselves, such as anger or guilt. Depressive feelings can take time to resolve but it is important to recognize that they can be treated and are a normal reaction to loss. However, if depression persists and interferes with other areas of your life, it is important to access help.

Depression can be accompanied by conflicting emotions that occur at the same time. It is common following bereavement or significant loss to feel sadness, anger and depression, all within a short period of time. Each day can feel quite turbulent when this happens. It can be helpful to talk to someone about this, as it may be the first time that you have experienced such confused feelings.

No matter what the circumstances of your loss, if you feel that you not coping well and are feeling increasingly sad and tearful, or are finding that you are tired all the time and lack energy, it is advisable to make an appointment with your GP, especially if you have had these symptoms for over a week. Your GP can give you short-term medication to alleviate the symptoms and assess whether you need additional support, such as counselling.

If you feel that your depression is acute or overwhelming, contact NHS Direct or Samaritans for advice and assistance. If you wish to have more specific support over the loss of a pet, contact the Pet Bereavement Support Service, run by the Blue Cross. Contact details of these organizations are given at the back of this book.

Grief and mourning

The way that we grieve is both personal and determined by social and cultural expectations. It is necessary to go through a period of mourning following a loss. This gives recognition to our loss and affirms the value of the pet we have lost. In some religions, there are set periods for mourning after bereavement that help to define the grieving, such as the Jewish *shivah*. At the end of mourning there is an implicit sense of completion.

It is often commented that as a society we hide our loss. You may find that, having lost a pet, you also felt the need to hide your loss, because you felt that you would not be taken seriously or you wanted to minimize the importance of the loss to yourself and others.

Our tears are an expression of our loss. Tears can come at different points in any loss process as we mourn what we have lost and the change that this brings. Many pet owners speak of the tears that come at the points of separation – at the vet's or at a cremation, for example. Afterwards, sorting out your pet's possessions can evoke tears. These are necessary tasks, however, and it is understandable to mourn this transition. Tears often come when leaving a familiar place, when we are feeling alone after the end of a ceremony, or having said goodbye to a pet.

Some pet owners find that the practicalities of euthanasia or natural death dictate a structure within which to mourn. From the loss itself to receiving the ashes back or a planned burial or personal remembrance service, there are chances to mourn that can be therapeutic in releasing feelings. Tears are a part of the process and are a natural human response to loss.

It is important not to minimize your feelings. Recognizing loss and the need to mourn is an implicit part of acknowledging your own needs. Sometimes it is not possible to achieve closure following your loss, but it is still possible to plan. One pet owner describes what happened after the death of her cat:

> When Bonnie died we had her cremated. I knew I wouldn't really stop grieving for her until we had decided what to do with the ashes. As we were moving in the next few months, we decided to keep the ashes so that we could take her with us in a way before scattering them in the countryside around where we moved. We like to think that she would have loved playing there, and it helped me to think we had taken her with us rather than leaving her behind.

Acceptance

The point at which you find acceptance following any loss is when it no longer burdens you. After all the feelings and emotions experienced after the loss of your pet you reach a point of reflection, when it is possible to hold memories without being troubled or distressed. You have accepted the limitations and the joys of pet ownership and the letting go that is eventually necessary. If this letting go has been sudden and traumatic, it has probably taken longer to reach this point than if you were able to prepare for it.

Acceptance may come long after you have got used to being without the pet, or when another has found its own place in your life.

But it is still important to have reached this point of acceptance with respect to the pet you have lost. Being able to reach acceptance indicates that you have found some kind of peace within yourself. This will probably have been difficult, demanding courage and self-acceptance.

Finding a sense of acceptance about what has happened will probably enable you to hold on to hope for the future, that the loss and grief that you have experienced has not left you unchanged. We all wish that any loss we have suffered will not have been in vain, that eventually it will leave us with hope. When facing uncertainty of any kind, we rely on hope to pull us through.

Helping yourself manage feelings following pet loss

Losing a pet affects people differently. You may not experience all the stages of grief outlined above. But we all react to loss, whether we show it to others or not. You may feel overwhelmed and distraught by your loss or you may be feeling resigned to it.

Grief reactions are defined by many variable factors. The following are some that could apply to you:

- Was your loss expected or was it sudden?
- Has your pet gone missing?
- Has the loss had a greater impact on you than you expected?
- Did you feel that you were persuaded into making a decision about your pet that you now regret?
- Are you experiencing this alone?
- Have you experienced a major bereavement of a spouse, partner or family member in the last two years?

As we have seen, many people find themselves feeling depressed and bereft after the loss of a pet. Depression shows itself in a number of ways and affects people differently. There is a difference between feeling temporarily low in spirits and suffering longer-term symptoms. Bereavement or loss can affect us deeply. It is important to be aware of how you are feeling so that if necessary you can help yourself. Attitudes to depression have changed considerably in recent times and there is now greater understanding of how personal losses can affect us.

If the loss of your pet has made you feel unhappy for longer than you had expected, or if other people are concerned about how you seem, the following signs may indicate that you should see your GP or seek some talking therapy:

- if you are finding it hard to concentrate
- if you have lost interest in activities that you usually enjoy
- if you feel that you have withdrawn from people around you
- if you find that you have not been sleeping well or have been sleeping too much
- if you are feeling bad about yourself
- if you have been crying a lot more than usual, or for a longer period than usual.

When and where to get help

It is advisable to get further help if you are experiencing distress that feels overwhelming and that will not go away. It is also advisable to seek help if you feel that you are unable to cope with your pet's loss. You may be particularly distressed if, for example, your pet has died as a result of a road accident, or as a result of a malicious action against either it or you. By actively seeking help, for yourself or someone that you know, you are helping the start of recovery.

The Pet Bereavement Support Service is one specialist organization that supports pet owners who are facing a loss or have experienced one. It is a national service and as well as running a telephone helpline, it can answer email enquiries and letters. Details are given at the back of this book.

If your feelings of loss and grief are persistent and are preventing you from managing your life as well as usual, or if you are experiencing sadness, it is again worth considering extra help. Some types of help are outlined below. The Pet Bereavement Support Service can also give you further information.

Counselling and psychotherapy

Having one-to-one counselling or psychotherapy sessions can be helpful when you are experiencing the stress of loss. As a general rule, counselling is short term and will focus on specific issues that concern you. If you feel that your reaction to the loss of your pet has been difficult to manage, then counselling can support you and help you reflect on why this experience has been difficult for you. Your difficulty may relate to other problems in your life, for example, or to previous losses.

Finding the right counsellor or therapist depends on a number of factors. Counsellors and psychotherapists follow a range of theoretical approaches according to their training and experience. You can obtain a list of registered practitioners from the recognized organizations, principally the British Association of Counselling and Psychotherapy and the United Kingdom Council for Psychotherapy. Their contact details are listed at the back of this book.

A number of GP practices now have counsellors and counselling is available as an NHS service. You will probably be offered about six sessions.

If you find that you are undergoing behavioural changes, such as anxiety or feelings of panic, following a loss then referral to a psychologist can be helpful. Using cognitive-behavioural techniques, where the aim is to change thought processes and behaviour in order to address specific problems, the psychologist aims to reduce or minimize symptoms and develop strategies that you can employ yourself if the symptoms arise again. Contact details for the British Psychological Society are listed at the back of this book.

4
Pet loss and children

When people look back on their childhood and the relationships that were important to them, they usually view their pets with particular fondness and affection. In childhood pets often become additional family members. Anyone who has had a pet in childhood will be familiar with the experience of bonding and the strong attachments to which this leads. For this reason, and because pet loss affects children in different ways, this chapter explores the importance of taking care when explaining pet loss to children.

Many parents think that witnessing the life and death of a small pet, such as a hamster, can be an opportunity for children to learn that life does not go on for ever. However, when faced with the reality of an ill pet that has noticeably changed in appearance and behaviour, your child may not have developed sufficient emotional resources or cognitive ability to make sense of what is happening. A pet's illness, even if expected, is often unpredictable. Children can become concerned and anxious at this. It is important to be able to guide them through the process so that it becomes less frightening and forms part of a wider understanding of life and death which will serve them well in the future.

The idea of death – of not being here any more – may trigger many feelings for all of us, but does so especially for children. It can evoke curiosity but also fear. It is your role as a parent to recognize these fears – to pick up on them when they are mentioned or expressed – in order to minimize the anxiety that your child may experience.

Witnessing the life cycle of a pet can be a significant point of learning, so it is important that illness and death as seen through the lives of pets are explained honestly. Modelling a sense of respect and care for pets, for their lives and their ultimate passing, can shape children's subsequent experience of loss.

It is also essential to be aware of the different ways in which children can misinterpret the meaning of loss. The loss of a pet who served as a confidante, stimulated a child's imagination or offered him or her the chance to take responsibility can be very hard. The psychoanalyst Elisabeth Kübler-Ross in her seminal work *On Death and Dying* comments on the way that children perceive loss: 'Death is often seen as impermanent, and therefore little distinct from a divorce after which [he or she] may have an opportunity to see a parent again.'[3]

This chapter will offer suggestions and draw from the experiences of others as a way of helping you explain loss to children. Of course, this will depend on the age of your children, the relationship that they had with their pet, the circumstances of the loss and your own beliefs. At the end of the chapter, I have also included some help for young people who may be leaving home for the first time and find themselves in the situation of having lost a pet, or of having to leave one behind. Whenever a child loses a pet, though, it is important to be as open and supportive as possible, so that your child learns that expressing emotion in response to loss is normal and healthy.

Tasks for parents

There are four main tasks that parents face when dealing with loss:

1 explaining how and why the pet has died
2 explaining what has happened to the body
3 supporting distress
4 putting the loss into some kind of perspective.

Explaining how and why the pet has died

The most important thing to remember when explaining about a pet's death is the importance of clarity and honesty. This does not mean going into excessive detail about what happened and potentially upsetting your child further, but it does involve explaining the death of the pet succinctly and truthfully. Children will know if you are not telling the truth, so avoid long-winded explanations that avoid the facts. It may seem easier to resort to euphemisms that make the reality seem cosier, but they invariably lead to confusion and the expectation that the death will not be permanent.

Be prepared for having to answer the 'Why?' question. 'Why did he die?' 'Why couldn't someone make her better?' 'Why did she die when she was only eight?' These are potentially complex areas of life and death. Don't be annoyed by such questions – it is a product of children's curiosity and their need to rationalize what has happened.

A good way to approach the subject is to link the loss with the child's observation of the pet over the past few weeks or months. If the pet has been unwell, it is more than likely that your child has noticed. She may have said something, or she may have said nothing and hoped that everything would be all right. Either way, being honest about the loss or impending loss is essential to avoid further grief later.

Explaining what has happened to the body

This can be the focus of fear, anxiety and curiosity, although if your child was fully involved in saying goodbye to the pet then the difficulty may be eased. It is best to be transparent about what has happened to the body; it is important to be clear and unambiguous.

If you decide to bury your pet in a garden, then the children can be involved in preparing a short service and in the planning of the burial. Children may wish to have their pet buried with a favourite ball, for example. Involving them in planting a tree or bush can also help. Burial enables children to have a clear, concrete understanding of what has happened, as they can see the body being lowered into the ground. Please note, however, that many councils have regulations about the burial of pets. It is important to check with the local council first.

If your pet is cremated then children can be involved in choosing what to do with the ashes. Again a ceremony can be planned in which the children play a part.

It is vital that this area is explained with sensitivity, as a child's bond with a pet can be such that there is anxiety about what happens to the pet after death. By being as clear as possible, you will minimize the taboo that can surround death and loss into adulthood.

Supporting distress

This is a key task following the loss of a pet. If you know that your child has had the chance to say goodbye and take part in the process of letting go, then the likelihood is that adapting will be easier. Of course, a sudden death will be more upsetting than one that has, perhaps through old age, been expected.

Boys and girls will frequently react differently, depending on their age and the circumstances. For example, boys may not want to admit to being upset if other people are around, but when on their own or when talking to you on a one-to-one basis they may more readily express sadness and become reflective.

It is easy to minimize the experience of pet loss, especially if the pet was old, or a seemingly insignificant creature such as a goldfish. It is important not to diminish the importance of the loss. Children may be capable of understanding that life does end for all living things. However, it may be the first time this has happened, so it is important to validate both your children's sadness and their curiosity. Acknowledge that they are upset about the death and that they have invested a lot in the pet through their lives.

Children also invest a lot in adults to guide them through experiences of grief and loss, so it is important that you acknowledge these experiences and do not diminish them. Advice to children to 'pull yourself together' can be damaging and have long-term consequences for a child's self-esteem.

Encouraging children to express their feelings is an important way to help them cope with stress after a loss. It is OK to cry; if this is how your child reacts, then it is healthy and should not be discouraged. Remember to reassure your children that although the pet has gone, you are not going anywhere and are still very much there for them. However, children should never be put in the position of having to support an adult in the same way.

Putting the loss in perspective

This can depend on your children's age and how receptive they are to looking beyond the grief itself. Older children may have more complex reactions to the loss of a family pet, as it will have links to their earlier childhood. There may be some denial too. If your child has lost a pet previously, then it can be possible to relate the current loss to a former one, but a child's first experience of loss will be difficult. The meaning of pets in your family, your experience and your interpretations all play a part in helping your child understand the loss. Photos and memories of happy times with the pet can be a good way of building up a picture of where it fits into your family history.

The first few weeks after a loss can be the hardest, as this is a time of readjustment for the whole family. It may only really hit home that a pet is missing when your child comes in from school and the pet is no longer there to be played with. Try to anticipate this by arranging other activities if you think it will help. This is not to avoid the reality of having to 'get over' the space that has been vacated by a missing pet.

Approaching pet loss at different stages of development

It can seem daunting to have to explain death to children. Our desire to 'get it right' can create anxiety for ourselves too, while our own ambivalence towards or fear of death can further complicate the way that we approach the subject. As adults we wish to protect children from painful emotional experiences, yet we also realize that it is important to tell the truth.

The age of your child will determine how he or she reacts to the death of a pet, and how you can best cope with this reaction. Approaching the subject of pet death with a child of two or three will be different from explaining it to a nine or ten year old. Consider the developmental stage of your child when thinking about how to manage the loss. The following general guidelines indicate how to approach pet loss with children of certain specific ages.

Two and three years old

Most children aged two or three will not understand what 'dying' means or fully appreciate reciprocal relationships – those that depend on interaction with other separate beings. The psychoanalyst John Bowlby claimed that children are able to establish reciprocal or two-way relationships from the age of three. However, just because they may not be able to rationalize what has happened or have a conversation about it does not mean that they will be unaware that something is different.

It is important to tell children even of this age that the pet has died and will not be coming back. They may consider the pet to have had a kind of sleep, but you should explain, clearly and unambiguously, that it will not be returning. It is best to avoid talking about the pet 'going to heaven' at this age, as this may set up the expectation that it will return, and the child will become confused or distressed when this does not happen. Even though at a conscious level there may be little understanding of death, there is the beginning of an understanding that life does not go on for ever.

This is where the lessons of loss begin. A child may not be able to articulate that the pet has gone but is likely to notice. He may be distressed and temporarily lose speech, so be sensitive to this. Likewise, at the age of two or three a young child will be able to accept another pet in place of the one that has died.

Four to six years old

By this age children will have a greater understanding of death. They may have heard or read stories that deal with pet loss in a matter-of-fact way. When faced with the death of a real pet, however, there is likely to be a sense of denial about the loss.

It is easy for children of this age to imagine that their pet is asleep somewhere and will be coming back soon, or that it is living with another family for a while. They may view the loss of the pet as being attributable to a number of things – being lost, staying somewhere else, living underground – and to imagine that it will return eventually to make everything all right again. When this does not happen, the sense of loss and disillusionment is intensified.

There may also be an underlying sense in which children blame themselves for something they said or did to the pet, or when the pet was around them. At this age children can invest a lot in the relationship that they had with the pet – its trust and security – and it is important that they know that it is not their fault that their pet has died or been taken to the vet to be put down.

There can also be a lot of fear around death and dying. Death holds a fear of the unknown and is still taboo even for some adults. If your child begins to communicate worry by a change in behaviour – such as bedwetting or waking up upset through the night – reassure her and encourage her to talk about her lost pet.

It could be that your child wants reassurance that nothing nasty has happened, that the pet is not in pain and that neither you nor the pet is cross or angry with her. Children may also need reassurance from you that they are safe; they may worry that because their loved pet has died they may die too. Grandparents, teachers and family friends can be valuable at this time in giving comfort and representing security.

It is better to talk to your children frequently in short conversations rather than holding long ones. This will mean that they are reassured at many different points and will be more likely to remember what they have been told. You could also involve them in the loss by having a burial in which they play a practical part.

If you decide to get another pet some time after the loss, be sensitive as to when you do it. There is a risk that it may lead to resentment or confusion about the new pet taking the old pet's place. Instead, introduce the idea of getting another pet and see how your child responds; this will mean that he has had a part in the process. The decision whether or not to get another pet is explored in more depth in Chapter 10.

Seven to nine years old

By the time children are a little older, the loss of a pet may assume greater significance but there will be less anxiety about the death itself. Children of this age will be able to separate the pet's death from any subliminal anxiety around their own mortality. Alongside a need to mourn the loss of the pet, there may be greater curiosity about the procedures that the vet will carry out and what will happen after the death.

Children of this age are likely to have a growing awareness of human mortality. They will have occasionally experienced the death of adults, such as grandparents or great-grandparents. The death of a pet may necessitate some reassurance about your own health and continued existence.

The death of a pet can feel like an abandonment. If your pet has been part of the family for as long as your child can remember, then its loss will be all the more significant. A child will often need to know that death is a part of the life cycle and that although we may feel abandoned, it is out of anyone's control. Reassurance should be given if the feeling of 'being left' is strong. Think about other recent changes in your child's life where he or she may have experienced loss – change of school, separation or divorce, or a close friend moving away. We can sometimes forget the bigger picture in children's experience. Loss happens in many ways through childhood and it is important to be sensitive to this.

Children at this age may seem as if they are coping but will show different signs of loss and grieving from younger children. Teachers need to be aware of any upsetting event, including pet loss, and how this can temporarily affect a child's mood.

Whereas a young child's reaction to the death of a pet may be quite spontaneous, when children grow older they may, for a number of reasons, take longer to react. This too needs to be taken into consideration, so that you do not dismiss the loss out of hand. Denial is a response that can indicate a wish that a major loss had not happened. It can provide a temporary suspension of the need to react, enabling the child to become used to the idea of the death. Yet when the grief reaction finally occurs, the child needs to be supported, and not diminished by stating that 'you should have got over that by now'.

Adolescence

For older children, those in and approaching the teenage years, a pet can still be a meaningful attachment figure. They are in the middle of a period of change that is often stressful, as they negotiate the path between childhood and adulthood. If a pet dies during a difficult point in adolescence, the loss can be experienced very acutely. Having a pet becomes a familiar link with childhood; during the difficult transition between childhood and adulthood, the family pet can be a link with the past, as well as a secure object of affection when no one else seems to understand.

Being confronted by the loss of a pet at this stage can feel overwhelming, but conversely it can be met with apparent indifference. It is important to be available to talk, while accepting that your child may prefer to talk with friends or others. You may think that the teenager appears to be indifferent to the loss but that does not mean that he or she is denying it.

Although it may not be 'cool' to grieve over a pet that was old or sick, it can accentuate an adolescent's feelings of isolation, so it is important not to ignore the effect that it can have. Peer support, the availability of trusted adults and the opportunity to talk are all important.

The influence of environment

In addition to their stage of development, children's experience and reaction to the loss of a pet will vary depending on the environment that they are living in. If you live in a rural area the loss of animals can be relatively commonplace and part of everyday life, especially in farming communities. Being near a variety of animals can give children the opportunity to hear about or even witness animal loss on a large scale. There is a greater acceptance of it, although even then there is likely to be a distinction between a family pet and other animals.

In rural communities, children learn early in their lives that the death of animals, for whatever reason, is part of nature and the environment. Some children will no doubt have been familiarized into this culture because of their community's involvement in hunting. Horses and ponies play a large part in the lives of many people, for example, as described in Chapter 1.

Children living in cities are unlikely to have been exposed to this culture and so will lack the same direct knowledge of animal loss. Although there are a number of wildlife and nature programmes on television focusing on animal issues, the urban experience is less immediately involved with animals. Therefore the knowledge may not exist to prepare such children when a pet dies.

Ways of explaining the loss of a pet

Whatever your children's age or situation, there are some principles to bear in mind when talking to them about the loss of a pet:

- Aim to be as straightforward as you can. This will mean that you will not become 'tongue-tied' or feel out of your depth. It is important that you feel confident in explaining things as clearly as you can, so that your child is helped to understand in a way that minimizes both their anxiety and your own.
- Use words and phrases that you know your child will understand. Don't introduce new words that may seem to be 'gentler', as you may get sidetracked into explaining what you mean rather than conveying the facts. Think about whether you are avoiding the subject for your own benefit rather than for the sake of your child. If possible, think about what you are going to say before breaking the news, as this will make you feel clearer about it.
- Choose a quiet space in which to talk. Background noise or leaving the television on, even with the sound down, will be a distraction.
- Explain that feeling sad about what has happened is normal. Be available to talk if your children wish to in the coming days and weeks, as this is all about modelling ways of coping with loss and stress, which are lifelong lessons. Do encourage feelings to come out following a loss – it is important not to discourage crying, no matter how 'big' your child may seem, as this is a valuable part of mourning.
- Do not lay the responsibility of telling your children about a loss on anyone else. As a parent, it is better coming from you, as you will be the one they trust. If you really feel unable to do it, involve another trusted family member.
- With older children, it may be useful to ask them where they think the pet has gone. This may facilitate a greater understanding of the unexplained nature of what happens when life ends.

Being honest

It is vital when explaining the death of a pet that you are as honest as possible. Some explanations, even though well meant, can be taken quite literally, especially if a child is young and does not understand the difference between life and death. Also, remembering that this may well be the child's first experience of loss, it is important to try and get it right. Anything that avoids the truth will cause problems later on and can be interpreted by children as a punishment or make them fear that they have done something wrong.

Losing a pet can damage a child's illusion that everything will always be all right. If this is the child's first experience of loss it is important that it is handled with care and kept in perspective. Losing a pet can be viewed as 'one of those things' that happens in life, but if this is the first bereavement the child has suffered, a lot of readjustment of her world view will be required.

Children invariably have lots of questions about what has happened. By involving them in the process and answering questions honestly you will be helping to build coping strategies around the inevitable challenges and disappointments that lie ahead.

Remember too that the loss of a loved pet can be an opportunity for a child to question many matters around life and death. There is a tendency for parents to wish to 'make things better' when approaching questions of mortality and to implement behavioural strategies to prevent avoidable distress. At the same time, however, the loss of a pet can be an opportunity for learning and developing a view of the uniqueness of life that can serve children well in their subsequent development.

Language

It is important to be straightforward and use direct, understandable language wherever possible. Consider the following statements which have been used to explain what has happened and the potential negative effect that they can have:

- **'Bruno wasn't well and so he went to heaven.'** This makes the connection between the illness of the pet and being in a safe place but it should be used with care. It assumes that 'heaven' is a safe place where nothing bad will happen. There is often no indication as to whether going to heaven is permanent. Nor does it indicate whether heaven is a real or an abstract place, so it may leave children who don't understand the notion of heaven feeling confused – especially if they expect the pet to return after it has finished its visit. The above statement may be suitable for use with a young child of two to four years, but should be used with care for older children.

- **'Bruno has gone on a long holiday so we won't be seeing him**

any more.' This may seem like a convenient way of explaining why the pet is not there, but it assumes that your child has noticed nothing about a pet's behaviour or any change in its health. It also runs the risk that the pet will be seen as having abandoned the family home because it didn't like living there or didn't like the people there. In addition, it may create anxiety about going on holiday and suggest a possible link between going on holiday and death/not coming back which may distress children.

- **'Bruno has gone to see Jesus/Allah . . .'** Although this can appear to be comforting, offering the idea that a greater or more holy or protective figure is looking after the now deceased pet, it creates the possibility of conflict. As well as being an abstract concept which can be difficult to define, it runs the risk of alienating your child from their existing belief or faith. Instead of being a source of comfort, it sets up a dynamic whereby the figure may potentially be blamed for the death. It is better to provide a more concrete understanding of what has happened.

- **'Bruno went to the vet's and they said he had to be put to sleep.'** This statement is based on what the vet may have said, but it potentially creates anxieties about sleep. What about when you tell your child to go to sleep? This can translate into fears about going to bed or having hospital treatment. It is better to let the vet explain that the pet's life has to be ended to avoid it suffering too much, linking this to behavioural changes in the pet that your child may have noticed in the last few months

Some people find it useful to explain the physical body as being separate from the soul or special part of the pet that is remembered. This can allow acknowledgement of the physical loss while enabling the child still to hold on to the special aspect of the pet, the part that connected with him or her. This is likely to fit in best with a religious belief system, but can also be more widely used in helping the child to hold on to the memory in a more tangible way.

Finally – it should seem obvious – it is essential to avoid linking the loss of a pet with a child's bad behaviour. If blame is attached to a death when we are too young to rationalize it or think it through, this can be massively psychologically damaging and can be destructive to a child's personal relationships with others. Blaming a child can have long-lasting effects and should always be avoided.

Above all, as stated earlier, it is important to reassure – especially if the sadness is felt by everyone – but also to validate the child's special connection with the pet.

Two case studies

Inevitably, the way that each person and each family deals with their loss is unique and is dependent on a number of factors. Grieving is affected by many things and will often not have a clear resolution. There is no textbook example of the right way to approach a child's loss.

Two brief case studies will illustrate this. The way you address pet loss with your children will inevitably be in keeping with the way you parent and will reflect the social and cultural traditions you are familiar with.

Case study: Elaine

Elaine had owned cats since before her daughter Jasmine was born. The family had a tradition of owning cats. Their present cat was Poppy, a neutered female now aged sixteen, while Jasmine was coming up to her sixth birthday. Jasmine had never known a time when Poppy wasn't there. Elaine had noticed that Poppy was getting far less energetic, passing urine a lot and becoming very thin.

While Jasmine was at school she took Poppy to the vet and it was confirmed that Poppy had severe kidney problems. Poppy did not regain consciousness from the anaesthetic but Elaine, although sad, was quite matter-of-fact about it.

Elaine's attitude contrasted with Jasmine's grief on hearing the news. At first Jasmine didn't understand, asking when Poppy would wake up and when she was coming back. It was when Elaine said that Poppy wasn't going to come back that she realized she could have dealt with things differently. She had not expected that Jasmine would be so upset.

For several weeks Jasmine's behaviour changed. She would cry when she came home from school and at one stage became angry with her mum, saying 'You took Poppy away.' Elaine felt very guilty when the strength of Jasmine's grief response became clear. After talking to Jasmine's dad and her teacher, and phoning the vet for advice, Elaine was advised to spend time talking to Jasmine about the reasons that Poppy had to go to the vet's. When she explained that Poppy had been 'put to sleep' (and what that meant) because she was so ill, Jasmine said she had noticed that the cat had been poorly.

Having talked about it over some weeks, Elaine came to understand Jasmine's feelings. When eventually they got another cat she involved Jasmine fully in the choosing of the new pet.

Case study: Yvette

Jermaine and Yvette had bought their son Junior, five, a kitten for Christmas. They had bought their daughter Avril a kitten called Polly for her birthday the previous August and as Junior had taken an interest in it they decided that it was a good time to buy a kitten for him too. The new kitten, Pushems, joined them on Christmas Day and was a great success. In good weather the two kittens went in and out of the house and appeared to be quite independent.

Sadly, Pushems went missing, having disappeared into a neighbour's garden. Yvette thought Junior was playing with him, while Junior thought he was inside with Yvette.

Although they put up notices in the local area, Pushems was not found. The stress of not knowing where he had gone was the hardest thing for the family. Yvette felt exceptionally guilty about what had happened and began to blame herself, as if by talking about it a lot she would make Junior feel better. Actually she herself thought she felt better by doing this, because she felt responsible in some way.

Eventually Junior told her at home that he didn't like to think about Pushems any more, and that he didn't want his mum to be upset any more. In effect this gave Yvette permission to stop mentioning it, but she did feel bad about reinforcing the memory and realized that she had been trying to sort out her own feelings of guilt rather than being constructive in the way that she supported Junior.

The above case studies show that there is no one way to support children when they lose a pet. In approaching such a loss it is useful to remember a number of things that help and others that do not. Those that can be helpful include:

- involving children in saying goodbye
- using play, art, photos and models to facilitate the narrative or story of a child's life with their pet

- being aware that children grieve in their own way and being sensitive to that
- having a memorial after a loss
- thinking about the role of the deceased pet in your child's life and beginning to reflect with them on the meaning of the pet in their lives.

Things that are not helpful and which are to be avoided include:

- imposing your feelings on a child, thereby confusing your feelings with theirs
- making assumptions about how they feel and what they want to talk about
- inhibiting any expression of the feelings that follow a loss
- talking about a replacement while there is still evidence of grieving
- presenting as facts things which are not true
- saying nothing and avoiding the subject.

When to protect children

There will be times when you will need to protect children from the circumstances of a pet's death. If the pet has been mauled or attacked by another animal, then this will inevitably be distressing. If they have witnessed this then obviously time should be taken to reassure them that this is not how animals usually behave.

Children will occasionally witness owners mistreating their pets. Again this can be distressing, as it will be outside many children's experience. All those involved with children should be alert to any claims that they make about animal cruelty, both in and out of their home, as this may indicate further abuse that could be affecting the children themselves.

Complicated grief

There are occasions when grief reactions in children are not straightforward and therefore need extra care. These are still losses but they need to be approached differently due to the circumstances.

Leaving a pet behind

If you are moving home, this occasionally necessitates leaving a pet behind, whether you are relocating to a different area of the country, into smaller or otherwise more limiting accommodation, or moving to a different country. Sometimes you may feel that your pet will have trouble in settling and you make the decision to leave it with friends. For whatever reason, it may just not be possible to take the pet with you.

In such situations it is important that you actively involve children in looking for a new home for the pet, so that they can be reassured that it is happy and settled. Explain to your child the reasons for leaving the pet – the practicalities of moving overseas, for example, or the fact that the pet would find it hard to adapt to a new environment. Use your children's knowledge of the pet to enable them to form a balanced opinion on the decision being contemplated.

The following points are important to explain to children:

- Tell them the reasons why you cannot take the pet with you. If the reasons do not seem legitimate, then this may make you reconsider. Think about it step by step. This will help you to recognize your reasons for a decision which will no doubt have been considered for some time.
- Remind them that neither your love for the pet nor theirs is in question.
- Remind them that your love for them is not in question.
- Finding a pet a new home is something that you are doing from a position of love, not anger or convenience. Stress too that they have done nothing wrong.
- Take care to recognize a child's fears about leaving a pet in someone else's care. Their relationship with the pet may feel irreplaceable to them, so be sensitive to the impact of what you are proposing. It can help to arrange a meeting with the owners to reassure your child of the pet's new home and safety.
- If your move is unavoidable and it is out of the question for the pet to come with you, try to create a situation where your child can play a part in the transition, either by visiting the pet in its new home or writing a letter to it explaining that it was not an easy decision to let it go but there was no choice. Thinking through the reasons why this is so will help your child to develop the tools to cope with all kinds of hard decisions around 'letting go' later in life.
- When a definite moving date is known, make sure the last few days and weeks are times when you can enjoy quality time as a family with your pet.
- Depending on your child's age, leaving a pet behind while

knowing that it is living somewhere new can be as much of a loss as any other and so should not be underestimated.

There have been changes in the past few years about pets being able to travel with you within Europe. This potentially avoids long periods of quarantine and means that pets no longer face months of separation from their owners. The PETS (Pet Travel Scheme) allows pets to travel with their owners through the use of microchipping. However, it does require several trips to the vet beforehand and care should be taken to ensure that all the requirements have been met. Contact details for further information are listed at the back of this book.

Missing pets

When a pet goes missing it can feel devastating. The initial shock and worry are replaced by what seems like a never-ending search. There is no guarantee that your pet will be found and this makes any resolution of the anxiety more difficult. Everyone who knows a pet that has gone missing will be involved in the process of worry. Helping children cope with this can be hard. Feelings of abandonment and guilt can be strong. 'Why did he run away?' 'Where is he?'

The topic of how to cope with missing pets will be covered in more detail in the next chapter, but for children it is important to:

- Tell them what has happened. Be open and honest. Hiding the facts will only make things worse and set up fantasies.
- Avoid talking about a return, as this will increase expectations that the pet will be found alive and well.
- Offer reassurance, particularly at night-time. Think of the missing pet as a problem that you are doing everything possible to try and sort out. Things like putting notices up and contacting the police reassure children that you are doing everything you can.
- Pick up on any expressions of guilt that your children may express so that you can let them know that it was not their fault. If it helps, encourage them to write a letter to the pet to express their feelings.
- If time passes and it feels right, plan a memorial service for the lost pet.

Hibernation

Some pets, notably tortoises, will hibernate for several months. When this happens, and if you are preparing the pet for hibernation, it is important to explain this to your child and to involve them in learning about how different animals function in different seasons. It is also wise to explain any potential risks and to minimize the risks that the animal is subjected to. One person I spoke to remembered the impact of finding that his tortoise did not 'wake up' from hibernation in the spring as it had been left in a place that was too cold. Having been completely unprepared for this to happen, he felt a huge shock and guilt at not being able to save his pet. If an adult had explained the risks and taken adequate care at the time, this distress might have been minimized.

'Taking in Granny's cat'

Sadly, there are times when an older member of the family dies, for example a child's grandparent or great-grandparent, and in addition to sorting out the estate of the deceased, there may be a pet to be placed. If this happens it can affect the whole family. Routines will be altered – if it is a dog it will need to be walked, while other pets may react warily to a new animal in the house. It is all too easy to neglect such responsibilities while the household settles into a new routine, especially if its human members are still experiencing sadness and grief.

Children in this situation are faced with a lot of readjustment. Even if they like the new pet, there is a risk that it may remind them about Granny's death and so act as a constant reminder, at least for the first few weeks, of what they have lost as well as what they have gained.

Conclusion

The way that each of us approaches the subject of pet loss will be different. With children, though, it is clear that it has to be treated very carefully because of the close relationships that children can have with their pets. Adults will remember the care and love that they were shown as children when facing a difficult transition and what can be an intense emotional and psychological loss.

For children the loss of a pet is not something that is simply read about in abstract through a textbook or story book, but will often be a tough learning experience. To recognize and respond to this is part of the wider responsibility that comes with parenting and child care.

To summarize, there are a number of things that you can do to help your child to accept the loss:

- Talk to them and answer as clearly as possible any questions that they may have.

- Pick up on anything that may indicate that they are worrying about what has happened.
- Hold a brief memorial service for the pet. This can involve reading a poem or story and maybe saying a prayer or giving thanks for the pet's life.
- Tell your child that they did not do anything wrong and that the death is not their fault.
- Do not make plans to replace a pet until you have talked to your child about it, and try where possible to include them in the decision so that you are all ready.

Losing a pet as a young adult

For thousands of young people, leaving home is an exciting time. Leaving childhood well and truly behind and moving to a new, independent stage of your life also means leaving your childhood pets behind. The cat you were given for Christmas when you were seven and he was a few months old is now eleven or older and coming to the end of his life. He is invariably left at home, as it seems unfair to uproot him from the environment where he feels safe and secure and where he is now looked after by your family.

You, in turn, will feel better that you have left the pet you adored as a child with your family, who can continue to look after him with the love that you once gave but now no longer have time to offer.

When a pet dies and you are away from home, it can bring special problems for you as a grieving owner. When you are given the news that your pet is dying or progressively ill, you may feel guilty that you were not there or powerless to know what to do. Losing a pet when you have only recently left home can be unsettling. Another link with your childhood has gone and any pet that your parents get as a replacement will be theirs, not yours.

What you can do if you are at college or university

- Tell someone if you are feeling sad and depressed following the loss of a pet. If your pet's loss has made you feel homesick, talk to someone rather than keeping such feelings to yourself.
- Talk to friends or tutors about the fact that you have experienced a loss, especially if you feel it is interfering with your ability to study and/or take exams. People will not know if you don't tell them.

- Recognize what your grief is related to. If you shared a close relationship with your pet through someone else – a parent or grandparent, for example, who has since died – it is understandable that the loss of your pet may take you back to a place of grief at a sadder time in your life.
- Talk to your college counsellor. Most colleges and universities have counselling services. If you are not at college or university but are still living away from home, contact your local library or look in the local phone directories for numbers offering counselling and psychotherapy services. Your feelings of sadness might not be recognized by everyone around you and it can be helpful to go to somewhere independent to talk about your feelings and loss.
- Do not blame yourself for not being there when your pet died. Recognize that you are at a different stage in your life now, which is a transition between your childhood and being an adult. You could not be at home when this happened.
- Keep a photo of your pet so that you can remember it when you are thinking about it.
- You may decide to get another pet when you are older and have finished college and keeping this in mind can help.

Signs that indicate you may be feeling depressed

If you experience one or more of the following symptoms following a loss, it is advisable to go and see either your GP or college counsellor:

- if you are finding it hard to concentrate a few weeks after hearing news of the loss
- if you find that you have lost interest in things that you usually enjoy and are feeling unusually sad
- if you feel you are becoming withdrawn, or people around you have noticed this about you
- if you are not looking after yourself, are eating too much or too little, or drinking too much
- if you are not sleeping well or are waking up at the same time during the night
- if you have started to take drugs or have increased your drug use
- if you have been crying for long periods.

Another good source of help is NHS Direct. See Useful addresses at the back of the book, or directory enquiries.

5

Missing: when a pet is lost

It is a fact of life that, unfortunately, our pets are vulnerable to going astray. Discovering that a pet has gone missing can be extremely distressing and may lead to intense feelings of anxiety. These feelings can increase as time goes on, if there is doubt about what has happened and the pet has not returned on its own. Having some idea of what to do if this happens can at least make you feel more in control. This chapter takes you through the steps to put into action if this happens.

Getting advice and informing the relevant people is essential. Contact addresses and website details are listed at the back of this book.

When a pet has run away

It is important to have an action plan so that you are able to follow things through step by step. The following initial steps are advisable:

- Check all possible places that your pet may be, for example sheds and outhouses.
- Ask local neighbours whether they have seen your pet.
- Contact the local police to see if any pets have been found.
- Contact local pet rescue services.

If your pet cannot be found after this:

- Design 'missing' and 'reward' posters to put up locally. If you are offering a reward for information or the return of your pet do not state a sum of money on the sign, as this may encourage false calls that may distress you further.
- Remember that taking action helps to contain your anxiety. It is important to remind yourself that you are doing all that you can.
- It may be that your pet has been temporarily taken in by a part-time owner who thinks that it is lost. Being able to identify your pet by means of a collar or microchip will make it easier for anyone who finds your pet to locate you.

Explaining missing pets to children

If you have children, especially those aged five and over, it is inevitable that they will notice that a pet has gone missing. While coping with your own distress and the panic that can follow on from the realization that your pet is missing, you will have to manage their distress too. It may be tempting to shield your children from any worrying change, but children are perceptive and even young children will probably notice very quickly when a pet is missing. Involving your children can be crucial to making this distressing time more manageable.

It is advisable to stick to the following guidelines:

- Do not keep the news of a missing pet from your children for too long. Tell them what has happened in a way that they can understand. They may have noticed and become distressed already, and it is far better to be open and honest. Hiding the truth from children can leave them with feelings of guilt and helplessness.
- Don't lull your children into false expectations of finding your pet if you don't know where it is. Saying 'We will find him/her' can set up an absolute expectation that the pet will be found when it may not be. Remember that pets are central to children's emotional lives and sense of responsibility.
- If there is a chance that your pet may be found, then say so and explain the different ways that this might happen, but be realistic at all times. If your pet has a habit of going off for a few days and then coming back, then link the disappearance to your experience of your pet's behaviour. But it is important to be honest at all times.
- Involving children in efforts to find a lost pet can make them feel that they are doing something to help. If your pet is not found, then it can comfort children to know that they were actively involved in trying to find it and did all they could to help.

Pet theft

Sadly, in the past few years the incidence of pet theft has increased considerably. It is extremely distressing when it occurs and results in massive anxiety for owners and pets alike. It feels like a violation and an exploitation of your attachment and love, as if someone you do not know has an utter lack of regard for you or your feelings.

On a recent radio programme about the subject, Tony Banks MP summed up the enormity of this situation by stating that 'having a pet stolen is like losing a member of the family'. Pedigree pets are especially vulnerable to theft, although pet theft in general has become more widespread. It is important to be realistic about the potential risks that are presented by people who are motivated by greed or by the desire to manipulate people's love and attachment to pets for financial gain.

Although it sounds as if it must be a criminal offence, there is no specific offence against 'dog-napping'; recorded incidents are seen simply as theft. Thankfully, in recent months there has been a good deal of publicity about this subject and the law may change.

At present there is no national strategy for co-ordinating animal theft, and the response to such incidents depends on individual police forces. However, there has been pressure within the government for legislation. There are also moves to improve communication between organizations such as the RSPCA, the Kennel Club, local authorities and councils.

There are some preventative measures that you can take to protect your pet from being vulnerable to theft:

- Try to be aware of where your pet is at all times.
- Avoid leaving your pet tied up outside public places where it is vulnerable to being stolen.
- Make sure that your pet has a collar and that comprehensive identification information is attached to it, along with your current address details.
- Have your pet microchipped so that it can be identified. Liz Emney from Battersea Dogs and Cats Home has confirmed that this is now a recognized deterrent against theft, and an asset if lost pets need to be reunited with their owners.
- Having your pet spayed or neutered acts as a preventative measure, because it then becomes less valuable.
- Consider taking out pet insurance so that you have financial peace of mind should anything happen to your pet.

What you can do

There are several formal steps you can take if you fear that your pet has been stolen or has gone missing:

- Contact your local police and give them full details of any

63

identification information that you have. However, you can only be allocated a crime number if you actually saw your pet being taken. The police will provide you with current advice on how to manage the situation if you are contacted or if a demand is made for the safe return of your pet.

- Contact the website <www.doglost.co.uk>. This offers support and advice and provides links with other facilities. By contacting them you will link into other services that can help you in the search for your pet.
- Contact Battersea Dogs and Cats Home. They have lists of all pets that are found.
- Be honest with children and do not attempt to hide the news of a theft. Involve them and reassure them about what you have done in attempting to recover the pet. It is important to stay positive when facing a worrying time.

Guilt and missing pets

Pets are fundamentally curious and, if able to do so, will go and explore their environment. Their curiosity, coupled with our inability to be with our pets every minute of the day, can lead to accident or theft, or attack by other animals. Your pet's instinct is to show independence, while your own instinct is to protect. Even with the best possible security, we cannot completely prevent accidents.

However, the sense of guilt experienced when a pet goes missing for no known reason can be powerful. We blame ourselves for something that is often out of our control. Even if the pet is independent and inquisitive, the feelings of guilt can still be strong. It becomes harder to rationalize a missing pet as being out of our hands or 'one of those things' if we feel responsible for its safety. We have traditions and expectations of how to care for our pets and there are social and cultural expectations of what we should do.

Our sense of not being able to control our pet's safety can lead us to feel powerless in the face of a missing pet. Yet we cannot know where our pets are all the time. It is unrealistic to know your pet's movements all day and night. All we can do is to make it as safe as possible for them. If our pets lived in a completely protected environment all of the time, that would take away their free spirit. An element of risk is essential to all life. Before it was common for people to have pets, they would be free to roam independently and take on that risk themselves.

It is important, while acknowledging the presence and origins of guilty feelings, to see them in the context of the degree of care that you showed to your pet. If you did not care then you would not feel guilt.

6

Accepting loss and grief

The quest to reach acceptance of your loss can take time and can be hard. There are ways that can help, but acceptance often comes after a period of mourning that can be intense and painful. Losing a pet that has been part of your life for some years can involve periods of doubt and exploration of your own identity and attitudes, and can be a long journey.

Finding meaning from your loss

We all have different ways of managing and justifying responses to loss. How we create meaning from our losses can be a positive indicator for readjustment. Having a consistent belief system that we apply to everyday situations can help us to move on from such losses. The interpretation of what has happened – the telling and retelling of the story – can help us to see things differently. This can bring a degree of comfort as we integrate our understanding of loss and gather new perspectives.

Many people are able to accept the reality of pet loss if they hold some spiritual beliefs. However, we would all wish to be able to hold on to hope after a loss, whether we have strong beliefs, are ambivalent or hold no beliefs at all. Without hope, losses feel more acute and there appears to be less chance of finding a way through.

Holding on to hope following loss

Although they may differ on many theological and ideological points, there is an appreciation of the importance of loss in all religions. Hope also lies in the belief expressed by many religions that the experience of bereavement and death brings us closer to a level of spirituality that is not always accessible to us. The death of a pet can focus our thoughts on notions of afterlife, or on holistic approaches to life, suffering and meaning. Most religions emphasize the sanctity of life, respect and the need for humane treatment of animals, and the importance of maintaining compassion towards all living things.

Animal psi

Pet owners often comment that they feel their pets understand them in a way no one else does. This is testament to the special relationship that is felt to exist between pet and owner. This relationship is personal and helps both during and after a pet's life. The degree to which animals are associated with myths and stories following their death may indicate our desire to believe in an afterlife where they are placed in a kind of collective unconscious to which we all relate.

The idea that there is some form of active communication – a psychic understanding that is more than conscious – enables many people to accept that in both life and death, something else exists. Of course it is difficult to prove that this kind of communication is real – it has often been dismissed as being unscientific and unproven – but there is a growing recognition of the part played by 'animal psi', as it is known. There have been numerous reports of changes in animal behaviour before natural disasters such as earthquakes. Animals are often credited with sensing catastrophes and changes in the environment or atmosphere that humans cannot detect.

One American parapsychologist, J. B. Rhine, researched the reported incidence of animal psi and concluded that there were several main types: animals were able to sense risk to themselves, to sense when their owner was about to return home, to be able to find the way home, and to sense when their owner was in some sort of danger.

Sometimes, too, people believe the spirit of their recently deceased pet remains around them in the weeks and months following their loss. This can be expressed in the form of the protection that they felt that was given to them. One owner said:

> Because she died so suddenly I felt in shock for a couple of weeks afterwards. Then, as I began to grieve more, usually on my own at home, I began to sense that she was with me, especially in the evening when I thought it would be worse. This went on for about two months. Then, as I stopped being so sad, I felt that she wasn't there so much – as if she knew I was all right now. But I do still sense her with me sometimes – just keeping an eye on me . . .

Personal grieving

Of course you may still want to mark the important place that your pet had in your life, even if you do not follow any particular faith or creed. This can offer a chance for reflection on what you think the important things are that have stayed with you through your journey. Holding on to these special memories can be comforting and calming as you begin to accept your loss. There are a number of ways to devise individual ceremonies after a loss or in remembrance that may be helpful to you.

Grieving for a pet shows itself in many ways and is different from other types of mourning. It is important not to put yourself under pressure to move on too quickly. Your loss was personal to you and is linked to a time of your life that you and your pet shared.

In the desire to end distress we sometimes try to hasten the end of our grieving, or we rush to find some meaning from the experience. This can take time. Give yourself time to recover. If you find yourself unable to do so after a considerable period of time, think about contacting one of the organizations listed at the end of this book.

Adults with learning disabilities

If you have a learning disability, you are more likely to experience isolation and find it difficult to sustain social relationships with people outside the learning disability community. Transition points in your life, such as moving from school to college or on to work or day care, can be stressful, confusing and often demanding.

You are likely to experience bereavement-like reactions to major life events, such as moving house or settling into residential care. And it is common for one loss to follow another. As well as moving home following a parent's illness or death, you may have to lose a relationship with a pet that cannot move with you. As an adult living independently, you may also experience an intense grief reaction to the loss of your pet.

Understanding the process of loss and illness can be made more real by the onset of illness in a pet. The reality of loss can hit home more powerfully when the pet you trust becomes ill and a decision has to be made to end its life. And facing the loss of a pet through natural causes can be just as stressful if there appears to be no clear reason why death has occurred.

If you are supporting someone who has a learning disability and who is distressed following the loss of their pet, it is important to remember the following points:

- Do not diminish the loss that someone with a learning disability may be experiencing following the loss of a pet.
- Involve the owner as much as possible in the options and choices available to them.
- Consider the life history of the person involved. If you are a carer who has been working with someone only for a short time, you will probably be unaware of previous losses, some of which may be recent and acute.
- If you are accompanying someone to the vet, ask them if they want you to come in to see the vet with you, but also be willing to wait if this is not what they want. Be prepared to support the person in asking questions.
- Explain matters of illness, euthanasia and natural death in as clear a way as possible. Try to explain in a way that is clear and unambiguous. Remember that if you are working with an adult who has a learning disability, it is important to avoid using childlike phrases or trying to 'make things better' by the use of euphemisms that may not be understood. If the pet has died or has to be euthanized, be open and honest about it and involve other people where possible, so that there is no mystery about where the pet has gone. The use of euphemisms actually causes more misunderstanding and confusion, and this will delay any grief reaction.
- Be prepared to support someone with a learning disability who has experienced a loss as and when necessary, rather than imposing a fixed timetable for 'getting over it'.
- Consider making referrals to local counselling/psychotherapy or psychology services, as the loss of a pet can evoke other unresolved losses. Any referral should only be made if the person involved gives their consent.

Helping someone close to you who has experienced pet loss

If you are close to someone who has lost their beloved pet, it can be hard to know what to do for the best. If you are not an animal lover but are concerned for the person who is grieving, here are a few suggestions that may help them to recover. Remember, it is not necessarily the size or type of pet that is important when understanding pet loss. It is the bond that has been lost that signifies the extent of the grief reaction. The following points may help at a time when it is difficult to know what to do:

- Take time to be with them, but also respect their wishes to have quiet time on their own if they wish to meditate or think alone.
- Be aware of any major changes in behaviour that could indicate depression or withdrawal.
- Encourage activity for part of the day to prevent them dwelling on grief too heavily.
- Encourage decision-making that will promote an active rather than a passive approach to the loss.

7

Pet loss in later years

Losing a pet when you are older can be particularly hard. By the time you are in your sixties, you will have experienced many losses and life changes. As people move into their later years, they make a number of choices about how they want their future to be. It is also the time when most people move into retirement. For many who have had busy lives outside the home, spending more time at home now seems both more feasible and also more appealing. It is a time to adapt and take on new interests.

Having a pet now becomes a realistic option, perhaps for the first time in many years. One reason that people often give when explaining why they do not have a pet during their working years is that there is not enough time to be with or exercise pets, particularly dogs. It seems unfair to neglect the animal all day when at work. But now, with more time available, many people find that having a pet around is a pleasure and offers a degree of companionship.

Today many people are living longer and more independently until their final years, while more people live alone in old age. This can be a challenge for some, especially for those whose family or friends live long distances away; our sense of community has changed in recent years as we lead more demanding and career-focused lives. For many older people this results in greater separation from those close to them and a reliance on pets for company.

Pet ownership becomes a part of life for many people in their later years for the following reasons:

- Having a pet may have been a part of their life for years, and having a pet in later years is part of a continuing tradition.
- Older people may have already experienced the loss of a spouse or of long-term friendships and find that having a pet offers extra companionship.
- As family and friends have moved away, there is more time to devote to pets and to value the relationship that they bring to life.
- For those who have experienced illness or reduced mobility in recent years, a pet can be company when they are at home.

Benefits of pet ownership

There are many benefits to having a pet in later years. Apart from offering company and a sense of belonging and being needed, they can establish a special place in your daily routine. They also offer the opportunity to establish emotional and friendship ties with others. Having a pet can be an instant talking point for people to share. The sense of shared experience and empathy with other owners can bring a greater connection to other people.

Pets can give a purpose to life when you have let go of other activities or they do not exist any more. Pets may come back into your life following a period of transition. The change from working life to retirement has already been mentioned, yet there are other transitions too – moving to a smaller house or flat can be made easier if you know that your pet is going to be moving with you. Moving to a different area or even just to a different house can be a major upheaval in people's lives, and pets can facilitate that transition by being constant and offering security.

Health benefits

There are many health benefits to pet ownership. These include lower blood pressure and reduced feelings of loneliness. Pets give people a reason to exercise and socialize, and give structure to daily routines.

Having a pet when you are older is an ideal opportunity for exercise, especially if you have a dog that demands to be walked twice a day. A dog could be said to be looking after you if you feel down or lonely by making you go out every day. A large number of studies have highlighted the health benefits of walking a dog, citing the lowering of depressive moods resulting from greater physical activity, a feeling of greater well-being from owning a pet and a lessening of the effects of cardiovascular diseases.[4] The action of stroking a loved pet can itself help to reduce stress and blood pressure.

One similar study compared adults before and after they had a pet and found a decrease in minor health problems among pet owners.[5] Another found positive indicators of morale and health for older adults living in the community.[6]

Pets can also be a reassuring physical presence. Having a pet in your home can be very comforting, especially if you live alone, and can increase feelings of security when you are alone at home. If you enjoy walking in the countryside or going for long strolls, having a dog can make you feel safe as well as being a great way to maintain your health and fitness.

Coping with loss

There are a number of reasons why it is important to consider the impact of losing a pet when someone is in their later years. Because having a pet has many benefits, it follows that the pain of losing a pet can feel more acute when you are older. Even if you have experienced a number of pet losses in the past, it can be hard when you have spent a lot more time with a pet around you at home to accept a loss as being 'one of those things'. The relationship between you and your pet is likely to have been strong as you invested more time with it and now miss your familiar companion.

If you had your pet for a number of years its loss can hit you particularly hard, especially if you have experienced a major life transition such as retirement. The time once spent with a pet can now feel empty, and you may feel a strong need to fill the space by getting another one almost immediately. Coping afterwards can be a problem, especially in the months following a loss. One pet owner in her seventies said:

> I thought I was doing very well after I lost Sheba. She had become a very important part of my life and I always imagined that losing her would be devastating. I think I managed well for the first few weeks because I knew why she had passed away. It was more in the months after that I really felt her loss . . . I found myself searching to know what to do with my time . . .

Coping with separation can be a problem even if the animal has not died. Another pet owner acknowledged that she found particular problems when she gave away some of her young puppies. Despite knowing that she would be selling them, actually letting them go became more of a problem the longer she had them:

> I have bred dogs all my life but have never really got used to the reality of giving them away. You cannot help but get attached to them and I have always found that to be difficult.

Financial concerns

One of the most difficult things you may have to face when you lose a loved pet is the financial cost of vet's fees. On top of the emotional impact that follows news of a terminal illness, having to find money to pay for treatment can add to your stress. There are a number of low-cost insurance schemes that can provide peace of mind. Alternatively, Age Concern can advise owners on what to do following the death of a pet. Their contact details are listed at the back of this book.

Above all, it is recommended that these things are planned in advance, so that financial worries do not trouble you unnecessarily. Having good, low-cost insurance and access to good advice can prevent stress at such times.

Replacing a pet

Whatever the circumstances of your loss, the relationship that you had with your pet will have been one that was unique and special to you. The risk of feeling isolated following the loss of a pet is real one, but it is important that you decide to get a new pet for the right reason. Allowing yourself time to mourn, and to recognize the unique relationship that has now passed, will ultimately make it more likely for you to form a new one. Each pet is unique and deserves to be seen as such in its own right.

Even if you decide not to replace your pet following a loss, or have one pet instead of two, nothing can take away the memory of your relationship with a pet and the part that it played in your life. People often associate particular stages in their life with what they were doing at the time. One 67-year-old owner was quite nostalgic when he talked about his life before retirement:

> Looking back on it, the time that he had with us was a happy time for him and for us. He used to love walking in the local park where we used to live. I remember before my wife died and our happy holidays with him.

You may feel that part of your past has gone with the passing of your pet. It is equally true to say that a new pet can be part of your future.

Following a loss it is understandable for a degree of apathy to set in when you consider getting another pet. Many people find themselves asking 'What's the point?', or not wishing to risk facing such loss again. If you are considering having another pet but are apprehensive about the emotional impact of further loss, the following points may be helpful:

- Make a list of all the positive and negative points of having another pet now. Maybe you feel that you are unable to offer a loving home to a pet, or do not wish to commit yourself to another pet at this stage.
- Think about getting a different type of pet if you feel that the energy involved in having another pet would be too much for you at this stage. It may be that a small dog is more suitable than a larger one or that a cat would require less of your attention.
- Consider your personal circumstances and what will suit you best, before acquiring and becoming attached to a pet that you would be distressed to lose if you had to let it go at a later stage.

What if I have to move into residential care?

If residential care is required it is frequently not possible to take pets with you. This is usually because of the individual care organization's policies. Out of 20 sheltered housing organizations contacted nationally, it was found that only two had any provision allowing people to keep their pets with them. Having to move is stressful at any time, especially if you are losing some of your independence. Being unable to take your pet with you can add to the feeling of loss and distress.

If this is the situation you face, it is worth planning in advance and finding a good home where your pet can be fostered, or a trusted friend or relative who can take it for you. Part of the care that relatives and friends can show at a time like this is to ensure the safety and happiness of a pet that may have to move to unfamiliar surroundings.

This remains a source of great sadness to many people who have to give up a pet in their later years. Many care homes are not currently able to offer facilities for greater contact with pets. Maybe as society changes and the demands of a growing generation of those over 65 assert their needs, this will be viewed differently and greater recognition will be given to the role that pets can play in positive psychological health.

Pets as Therapy is an organization that provides regular animal visits to care homes for the elderly. It aims to provide a link between people and pets when it has not been possible to maintain such relationships. Their details are listed in the back of the book.

Relatives and friends

The role of relatives and friends can become increasingly important as people move into their later years. However, if it is known that someone has a pet it can be used as an excuse to not contact a relative: 'They're all right – they have their dog/cat for company.' A pet can indeed be good company for many people but should not be used as a substitute for personal contact.

Likewise, if you know someone who has recently experienced the loss of a pet, be aware of the effect that this could have on them. The following points are important to bear in mind:

- Don't underestimate their loss. It could be that the loss of the pet feels devastating to the owner and that he or she needs your support. You may have to be the one to get in touch, rather than relying on your friend or relative to do so. People facing grief often wish to 'hide away' from others, especially when facing personal distress.
- Don't ignore signs of depression – a period of feeling low may be understandable following the loss of a loved pet, but if this continues for a long time it can be difficult to move on. Be available. Be supportive.
- Avoid rushing in to get a replacement pet if it is clear that grief is still active. Take time to talk about what the owner wants. You could be assuming that they want another pet when they don't. Imposing what you feel is best for them is not always helpful.

Preparing for your pet's future

Many people make provision in their will for what will happen to their pet and are obviously concerned for the pet's future and security. Knowing that your pet will be well looked after is a source of comfort. If you are a relative or carer for someone who is facing rehousing or a terminal illness, it is important that you respect their wishes and do not underestimate the importance of this task.

If this is something that concerns you, think now about what you would want for your pet. It is easier to make such decisions in advance so that they do not trouble you later. Doing some research now about the options can be reassuring and put your mind at ease.

8

Losing a service dog

'A guide dog is almost equal in many ways to giving a blind
man sight itself'
  – Musgrave Frankland, one of the first people in the UK
to have a guide dog in the 1930s

The unique relationship that people share with their pets has already
been explored in this book. Losing a service dog can be especially
difficult. The way that guide dogs are trained, placed with owners and
then retire means that there is a definite beginning and end to this
working relationship, requiring owners to manage the separation.

Examples of the helping relationship between dogs and people
have been documented for hundreds of years. This unique relationship was depicted on murals found in the ruins of Roman
Herculaneum. In the aftermath of the 1914–18 war in Europe, dogs
were used to help soldiers who had been blinded by poison gas, and
their success in rehabilitation indicated that the idea could be
widened to help those with existing visual disabilities. Subsequent
developments in other countries led to more research, and now guide
dogs are an option for blind and partially sighted people worldwide.

Losing a service dog through retirement or hearing news of its
later death can be extremely upsetting. The degree to which there is
a continued relationship with the pet after it retires can affect the
intensity with which the loss is felt. After retirement the dog may be
kept as a pet or rehomed with a volunteer. Some people decide to
have no contact after the dog leaves, but the impact of separation
still has to be considered.

Helping to develop the bond

Having a guide dog offers its owner freedom and increased
confidence. The high intensity of training when a dog and owner are
first brought together can forge a mutual dependency and attachment.

Selecting the right dog for the right owner is a task that requires
skill and experience on the part of the placement worker. There has
been a degree of matching already in assessing compatibility of

lifestyle, height and stride, but the bond between dog and owner really begins at the point when a selection is made. The two are then at the start of a working relationship that can last for a number of years. It is inevitable that the interdependency between dog and owner will be a key factor in the success of that relationship.

If you have a guide dog, or know someone who does, you will be familiar with these issues. However, if this is your first guide dog then it is important to discuss this with your placement worker. Losing a dog at retirement can be a difficult separation; knowing that the working life of a dog and therefore its time with you is likely to be limited will help you to be realistic, and to prepare for that separation.

Accepting when it is time to let your pet retire

It would be wrong for a working dog to have too long a working life. The average working life of a guide dog is about seven years, and knowing this should help to prepare you for the time when your dog is due to retire. This still does not account for the emotional pull of separation when the time comes, however, especially if it is decided that your dog is going to retire away from you. In these circumstances it is important to try and remember:

- that there is a limit to a dog's working life
- that your dog will be looking forward to a happy retirement
- that the organizations that placed your dog with you are available for consultation throughout the process
- that if you have had previous experiences of this kind of separation, it may be useful to draw upon what helped last time.

Starting the process again

Your placement worker will help you to begin life with a new dog. He or she will be familiar with the process of transition and bonding that needs to happen when a new pet and owner begin their life together. One owner said:

It helped me to have regular contact so that I knew that I had someone who would be able to guide me through when Lucy retired and while I was getting used to Freda . . . I know that I get attached to my dogs and being encouraged to think ahead about the changeover to a new pet helped enormously.

It is probably helpful to go through this period of transition by taking one step at a time and keeping in regular contact with your placement worker. Bonding with a new dog is likely to take some time and it is important to get the bond right.

News of a death after retirement

It can be sad to hear of the death of a guide dog with which you had a bond for a number of years. Hearing about it from a distance, after the animal has left you, may give you a sense of loss and regret. You will have said your goodbyes, but the death can bring up unresolved sadness. However, many past owners whose dogs have retired take comfort from the knowledge that the dog had a well-deserved and rewarding retirement.

Having said goodbye at the end of the working relationship, it may help to view the passing of a retired guide dog with regret, but also as one would an old friend who has been distant for some time. Giving thanks for the special time you spent together can be a fitting tribute to what was a valuable bond.

Hearing dogs

Just as a guide dog can be a vital link for blind people, dogs have proved to be successful in enabling deaf people, or those with significant hearing loss, to be more independent. Training is given to selected dogs who are then placed with deaf owners. There are currently about 800 hearing dogs placed in this way and the annual placement rate is about 150.

Instead of responding to spoken demands, a hearing dog responds to other cues such as hand signals. Dogs are also able to notify their owner of sounds around them that facilitate communication. Having alert responses is vital in enabling an owner to minimize risk and maximize independence, highlighting sounds such as the doorbell, telephone, smoke alarm or other unusual noises. A hearing dog can add to its owner's confidence when living independently.

As with the loss of a guide dog, losing a hearing dog can be upsetting. Beyond the loss of the actual pet there is the loss of a relationship built on trust and reliance, and which has offered an owner a gateway to increased independence. Claire Guest, from Hearing Dogs for Deaf People, says that the process of losing a hearing dog is different from that of losing a guide dog. This is mainly because hearing dogs have longer working lives. Whereas guide dogs tend to retire after about seven years, a hearing dog can be with its owner for much longer.

It is usually evident when a hearing dog is at the end of its working life. It may be apparent at the animal's six-monthly check-up and is indicated by its slower responses to sounds. If the dog sometimes 'opts out' or misses out on certain key sounds, then this can indicate that there is a deterioration in its alertness and ability to hear the necessary cues for its owner's safety or awareness.

Typically, the older hearing dog will continue to live with its current owner rather than retire away from him or her. At the same time, a younger trainee hearing dog will work with the owner. Many deaf recipients opt to keep their old dog as a family pet and it spends its final years with them.

Losing a former working hearing dog can be upsetting, especially as the bond will remain strong with the owner through the pet's life. If you, or someone you know, has lost a hearing dog, contact the link worker for further advice. As with other losses, it is important to give yourself time to grieve and for others to recognize your loss. The contact details for Hearing Dogs for Deaf People are listed at the back of this book.

9

Remembering a pet

The memories that we hold are a vital connection with the past. They offer hope of a continued relationship of sorts with the pet that we have lost. The way that we remember is also an opportunity to interpret and reconstruct relationships without having to let grief dominate. As mourning passes and we begin to be reconciled to the loss, there is a chance to reflect. This allows us to see things differently. While, following any loss, we cannot change the facts of what happened, it is possible to re-evaluate how it is seen.

Our feelings towards the pet that we have loved and lost may change as time moves on and our perspective alters. It may feel as if we are looking at things in a different way and this can seem unfair to the pet that you have lost. You have the luxury of being able to change your perspective on what has happened, whereas your pet does not. We can sometimes feel guilt when reinterpreting and evaluating the relationship we had with a pet, especially if, with time, we see it in a more negative light or think we might have done things differently. Ultimately, though, viewing your loss differently over time can be an opportunity to give thanks for the relationship and bond that you shared.

Putting grief in context

As time passes, it is usual for the grief we feel to begin to diminish. One of the gifts of time is its ability to allow us to put bereavements and losses into some kind of context or perspective. Over the weeks and months following a loss, this allows us to distance ourselves from the pain of separation. Obviously the degree to which this happens will depend on the circumstances of the loss. It is important to remember, however, that loss is part of a process. Your memories and reflections on your loss will change over time.

Doubts

After a pet has died it is understandable to continue to hold doubts and questions. We may question what happens to the soul or spirit of a pet, or whether we did the right thing in allowing a loved pet to leave us. This is unique to pet ownership, for as humans we can decide when a pet's life is to end and are able to make informed decisions about this. Having made these decisions, however, when reflecting on your pet's life it is important to remind yourself of why they were made.

If you feel that doubts are getting in the way of your grieving and are being translated into feelings of guilt, then remind yourself of the reason that you acted as you did and that it was in the best interests of your pet, so that you prevented it from further suffering.

Your doubts may be reduced only as time puts your loss into context. A sense of perspective often comes with the passage of time and makes our doubts easier to tolerate. One owner stated:

> It was only after about six months without Boxer that I came around to feeling that I had done the right thing. If he had still been here – and that is very unlikely – he would have been in even more pain and I wouldn't have wanted that for him or me. It was hard but now I think I did the right thing.

Having put most of your doubts to one side, it becomes easier to remember your pet in the way that you would want to. People often find that over time, memories give them new perspectives on loss, as if they can reframe the relationship they had in a different way. This can be one of the gifts of time, allowing us to cope with pet loss more positively.

Dreams

Our dreams can say a lot about our psychological states and are particularly relevant to the processing of loss and grief. Dreams can enable us to access more primitive parts of our mind. They can also be explored as being representative of the way we are processing our loss.

Caro Ness in her book *Secrets of Dreams* suggests that the appearance of a dog in your dream can be about loyalty and friendship.[7] Dogs also represent our masculine side, and a dream about a dog could indicate that we should channel things that are making us frustrated into positive ways. Cats, on the other hand, are seen to represent our feminine side. Domestic cats that appear in dreams can be about how we perceive our role in society: cats are naturally wild, but, like many people, have to conform to what is expected.

If you have dreams that distress or worry you following your pet's death, they are likely to be related to your unresolved 'searching' (see Chapter 3). Alternatively, dreams can be a way of processing unfinished anxieties. Such anxieties may not present in dreams in a regular or expected pattern. If you find that your dreams are worrying you rather than being of comfort, then it may be worth considering counselling or psychotherapy to throw some light on why these concerns are presenting now.

Ways of remembering

Planning a ceremony of remembrance can be an important part of your grief process. It gives you the opportunity to acknowledge your grief, whether you do this on your own or with other people present.

Despite all the loving care shown by your vet and the staff at the surgery, if you have a small pet at home or if you are faced with acknowledging that your missing pet is not coming back to you, it can be helpful to hold a ceremony. Planned when you feel it is right, this can be immensely healing. It gives a focus for grief that you can look back on. You can dictate what you include and where it will take place.

Having a ceremony of some kind can also make your loss more real. When we are moving towards acceptance, whether we believe in a continued existence or not, it is part of our ongoing denial to try to push away what has happened almost as if nothing has changed. Looking back on a ceremony can reassure us about the relationship's importance.

Cultural and religious beliefs are frequently integrated into the form and content of remembrance. It could be that your pet has represented a part of your culture and that in the ceremony of remembrance you are able to integrate customs that are important to you and your memory of your pet. Our past and present experiences can dictate when and how we celebrate life as well as how we mourn passing.

Planning a ceremony

It is important to try and plan the ceremony in advance so that you will know what you want to be said or done. During times of grieving, knowing what will be done or said at a ceremony can give us a greater sense of control at a time that can feel distressing and upsetting. The comfort of ritual – of making the ceremony as personal as you can to reflect your pet's life and your memories of it – can be calming.

Ceremonies can involve readings, prayers, candles, photos and personal momentoes that were part of your pet's life and reflect its uniqueness. A ceremony may remind you of past losses, or of associations that your pet had with loved ones who are no longer there. Try to think ahead, so that you are prepared for such memories when they come back.

Some ceremonies are focused on a pet's ashes. Taking these to a special venue or scattering them in an area that was personal to you and your pet can be very healing. Above all, by planning a ceremony that you are comfortable with, you are doing yourself and your pet justice by honouring its life and your connection.

Mementoes and memories

As well as planning a ceremony, thinking about what you wish to do with your pet's belongings can bring a degree of comfort. These can be extremely evocative of your lost pet, so it is wise to take time over this. Being able to decide what to do with its belongings is part of the grief and process of letting go, and can also leave you with the feeling of being in greater control in a difficult situation.

One person I spoke to in the course of researching this book had decided not to get another pet, but took comfort in giving away the personal effects of his dog. He spent some time deciding who to give the basket to, then the dish, and so on. By recycling some of his pet's effects, he felt that he was continuing to recognize the part that it had played in his life.

Greyfriars Bobby

Of course, it is not just humans that remember pets. The story of Greyfriars Bobby illustrates how pets can also grieve for their owners.

In 1858 a man called John Gray was buried in Old Greyfriars churchyard in Edinburgh. The grave had no stone to mark it and was soon unrecognizable and unnoticed. However, Gray's faithful Skye terrier had been so devoted to him that he kept watch over the grave for years afterwards. His devotion was recognized by local people and when the dog himself died, it was decided to put up a monument to commemorate the relationship between the two. The statue in Edinburgh is a testament to the bond between man and dog.

Keeping memories alive

There are many ways that you can keep memories alive and this can be a comfort as you reflect on the loss of your pet. Following a loss, especially soon afterwards, it can feel too painful to think about your pet. Coming home to an empty house, missing the familiar tap of paws on the floor, can seem to magnify the loss.

If you can, however, find ways of keeping your memories active they can be reassuring and comforting to you. Even if you decide to get another pet, however long afterwards, nothing can take away the special memories of your previous pet. Special days or anniversaries can be opportunities for remembering and can provide enriching memories.

The memories our pets leave us with are their legacy to us. Remembering is our way of keeping these legacies alive. No one can take away from you the memories that defined your relationship with your pet and the times you spent together. You may find that the time you had with your pet will spread across other major events in your life and can be especially poignant because of this.

The desire to 'do something'

Following the loss of a pet, some people find that they want to be involved in an activity that involves them having contact with other pets. Helping out at a local animal centre or with a pet organization is one way of doing this. Alternatively, doing voluntary work at a local animal charity shop can put you in contact with others. Taking a positive step to do something different arising from your loss can be very rewarding. It also means that you can construct further meaning from your experience.

Finding calm

As time moves on it is probable that you will be able to put your experience into some kind of perspective and find calm through the actions that you have performed to remember your pet. Remember that a pet's loss is not your fault. Life for all living things is ultimately limited. Caring for pets is a significant responsibility and one that we carry with us. By honouring your pet's memory in the way that you feel is right, you have done all you can.

10

Deciding about another pet

If you have lost a pet, it is understandable to have strong feelings about whether or not to bring a new one into your home. Equally, many people are unsettled when trying to decide what to do. This reflects the reality of pet loss, and the subsequent decision about acquiring another pet can be difficult to resolve. It can be hard to welcome another pet into your home if you have not worked through the previous loss or are still suffering feelings of guilt or regret from your last experience. It may take only a short time to recover from the sadness of losing a pet, or it may take much longer. Each experience is different.

This chapter aims to help you to look at the questions and feelings involved in getting a new pet. Whether you are acting on your own or as part of a family, everyone will have a view on what you should do. Above all, however, it should be your decision, so that you can take responsibility about what you do.

Thinking about getting a new pet can bring up many conflicting feelings about your future. Your recent experience may lead you to anticipate suffering a further loss. Alternatively, you may now be at a new stage in your life and have to think about other things that could influence your decision. If other people are suggesting that you have another pet, remember that the outcome of the decision will affect you more than anyone else.

There is no pre-set formula that will determine if or when you should make this decision. The reality of adjusting to a new pet can be hard for some, welcome for others. Whatever you decide to do, bringing a new pet into your home following a previous loss is a time of transition for both you and your pet.

Most of all, it cannot be taken for granted that welcoming a new pet in your life will 'solve' or take away the grief that you have experienced. In *Pet Loss: A Thoughtful Guide for Adults and Children*, Neiburg and Fischer state:

> Stifling one's emotions by investing energy and love in another pet does not eliminate grief; it merely pushes it into the background and delays its resolution. The sense of loss may take years to dissipate – or it may never disappear.[8]

Take care how you introduce a new pet to a household that still maintains memories of the recently deceased pet. Ask for others' opinions about welcoming a new pet, be sensitive to the emotions of children in your family, and try to anticipate any behavioural reactions that other pets may show by introducing the new pet gradually.

Letting go of your past loss

One of the main reasons people decide to have a new pet is that they have had a positive experience with their pets in the past. If having a pet has enriched your life, then it follows that having another is likely to do the same. However, this can only be done if you have 'let go' of the deceased pet. It can take time to get used to the space left by a pet who has passed away. The emotional bonds are still intact, even if the physical ones have been broken. Our attachments to pets do not fade and there can be unresolved feelings of grief if a pet who has recently died is still in our minds.

Remember that your bond with your pet was special and unique to you. The history that you shared, the way that you were witness to your pet's life at different stages, and the way that it was witness to a part of your life too are all important to recognize. Acknowledging these points is essential in beginning to accept the loss; if there are feelings that you are repressing it may be a sign that you have not yet accepted your loss, and this may prevent you from making a decision about having a new pet.

At this point it can be helpful to talk about your loss with a friend who knows you well, or with a professional counsellor. A friend may be able to offer a listening ear, and having known you for some time, may help you to make your mind up about what to do. As long as he or she does not push you into making a decision or unduly influence you, this is helpful.

Talking with a trained counsellor can help you to think about the loss that you have experienced following your pet's death. It is often a good way to talk about and explore your grief. Many people find that talking to someone who is impartial and who will be non-judgemental helps them to accept the loss. If the loss of your pet has taken you back to other unresolved losses, then counselling is helpful here too. (See the section on counselling and psychotherapy on p. 40, and the addresses at the back of this book.)

Questions to ask yourself

It is worth asking yourself the following questions when you are thinking about having a new pet:

- Have you resolved the loss of your previous pet sufficiently?
- How would having a new pet with different demands and more energy affect you?
- Is this your decision or are other people putting you under pressure to have (or not to have) another pet?
- If this pet is going to be a member of your family, does everyone agree about having a new pet?
- Have you agreed that everyone will share some responsibility for caring for the pet, or is it likely to cause conflict in the family when only certain family members do this?
- Do you feel that since having lost your pet, your life has been empty and something has been missing? Are you ready to take on the responsibility of a pet again?
- Are you likely to be moving home in the next few months?
- Did you have a very strong attachment to your pet which will make it harder to think about accepting a new one?

Dealing with ambivalence

If the questions above made you think that there may be some indecision or doubt about having a new pet, or have made you uncertain about what to do, it is likely that you are still holding some ambivalence or conflicting feelings. This often stops people from making clear decisions, and can sometimes make grief last longer, as you may want to move on but are not ready.

It is best to take your time if uncertain what to do. Making the wrong decision at the wrong time or acting too soon can have negative consequences and may lead you to regret your decision.

The loss of a pet can confront us with truths about ourselves or our previous feelings. Recognizing these mixed feelings can be hard and make us feel guilty, sad or angry. Looking back, you may feel that you never actually wanted a pet at all – that you were the one that always had to look after it, pay the bills, stay up all night when it was ill, and so on. In short, some people do feel, looking back, that having a pet was, on occasions, a burden, and that having another pet would commit them to further tasks that they are no longer willing to do.

It is true, however, that while some people see the responsibilities of pet ownership as a burden, others see them as a joy. It is important to recognize how you feel about this when considering whether or not to get another pet.

If a pet was given as a gift, then this too can create mixed feelings if it dies. Although the gift was welcome and the pet had a happy and contented life with you as the owner, you may be reconsidering whether you wish to replace it. This may necessitate tactfully telling anyone likely to give you a replacement that you have decided against another pet.

When feelings, commitment, emotions and history are involved, it is always easy to feel as if you are reaching no conclusion. Thinking more specifically about what you want and what you are able to give can help to determine what you do.

For and against getting another pet

The following are some factors that may help you to decide whether or not to invest emotionally, physically and financially in another pet.

Positive factors

- Finding company again. It is common for pet owners who live on their own, either through choice or following a loss or separation, to experience a sense of loneliness when their pet dies. Having been directly involved in the loss of your pet, you will also have been intimately involved in the physical loss of the bond between you. Having a new pet can bring another life back into your home.
- Giving you security. Pets, dogs in particular, are good at making us feel secure. The presence of a dog in the house at night can indicate if there are disturbances and reassure us that we have more, not less, reason to feel safe. Dogs can also give confidence to people when out walking; they give an added sense of protection as well as a focus for friendly conversation with other pet owners.
- Touching and stroking pets has been found to be very therapeutic and calming. Having a new pet may take some time to get used to, but will eventually serve this function. If your last pet enjoyed being touched and stroked, then it is likely that you will want to choose a type of pet that will do the same.

- If you have had a tradition of keeping pets, then after some time you are likely to be ready to continue this, and will be interested to see how your new pet is similar or dissimilar in personality to your previous ones.

Negative factors

- Not wishing to experience another painful loss. You may feel that the upset that you have suffered in losing your last pet has been too much to go through again, especially if the loss was comparatively recent. If so, remember that there is no rush and that you can always put off this decision until you are ready.
- Financial. You may feel that committing yourself to the cost of another pet is beyond your means at present.
- Your lifestyle and routine may have changed so that it is not so convenient to have a pet any more.
- You may need more time if you are experiencing unresolved grief and/or feelings of guilt.
- Adapting to a new pet with a different personality can be quite a challenge. If you are wondering about this, check out the pet that you are about to take on and if possible spend some time with it, either for a short stay or visit, to see if its temperament is compatible with yours. After all, having a pet is a commitment that will potentially last a number of years, and it is important for both the pet and you to feel comfortable.

The following case studies illustrate some of the factors that should be taken into account when we consider replacing a pet:

Case study: Alice

Alice, 78, was devastated when Portia, her Persian cat, was diagnosed with the advanced stages of leukaemia and had to be put to sleep. Portia was only four years old and Alice could not believe it when the vet gave her a terminal diagnosis. Portia had originally come to Alice through Eileen, a friend of Alice's niece, who knew a local Persian cat breeder. For the past four years their routines had been intertwined. Although Alice had been living on her own for some years, she did experience spells of loneliness. Having a cat seemed the perfect solution, providing Alice with company and the sense of being needed. This had been behind her niece's intention, as she had been concerned about her aunt becoming lonely.

91

Portia's passing seemed so sudden and unexpected. Alice felt bereft. She had lost her routine, her company and her reason for getting up each morning. The bond between the two had been established very quickly and when Alice went out to the local shops, people would usually ask her how Portia was. Portia had become part of Alice's identity and she felt that part of herself had gone. From being needed to being in a position of mourning and feeling lost was very hard indeed.

In addition, Alice didn't know how to respond. It had been years since she had a pet. There was no pre-written script on how to respond in this situation.

For some weeks, Alice's niece was increasingly concerned about her. She felt responsible for her aunt and began to regret getting the cat in the first place, as it had brought about this unexpected loss. She was not a cat lover herself and did not know what to do. Eileen had heard about Portia's death and contacted Alice. Within a week she had arrived at Alice's home and presented her with Bonny, a slightly older tabby cat that needed a good home.

To begin with, Alice was unhappy. She still missed Portia, and resented having to look after a cat that she felt wasn't hers and wasn't anywhere near as loving as her recently lost companion. She still had to feed Bonny and for a while it seemed that the new cat was a constant reminder of Portia. Over the next few months, though, she got used to Bonny's presence. She was never a replacement for Portia, but she still had to be looked after, and this gave Alice a sense of being needed.

Case study: Raj

Raj, 35, divorced three years ago. The dog, Buster, whom he had chosen together with his ex-wife but with whom Raj identified more closely, had come to live with him in his new flat. Following the split from his wife he found that walking Buster had continued to be part of his daily routine as before. However, there were also times when he had to take Buster to the kennels, either when he went on holiday or when he felt tied down by the routines of walking and feeding him.

As Buster grew older and became less mobile, Raj became increasingly aware that owning a dog was a large commitment to carry alone. He felt guilty that he could not spend more time with Buster, especially when he was out at work during the day. As

Buster came to the end of his life, Raj found that the emotional effect was hard to bear. When Buster eventually died, Raj felt a mixture of sadness and relief.

His immediate thought was that he would replace Buster with another dog, perhaps a puppy, but ultimately he decided to wait for a while. After a few months, his work and social life picked up following a promotion and, partly through commitments, partly through choice, he found he was usually out for at least four nights a week.

In the end Raj decided not to have another dog, as he felt that he would be unable to give it the attention and exercise it needed. Although there were times when he missed the companionship of a pet, he realized that now was not the right time for one, although he would reconsider if his situation changed so that he was at home more. The bond he had with Buster belonged to a time when he was feeling low following his divorce and he now felt he was moving into a different phase of his life.

Several key points arise from the above cases:

- Deciding whether or not to have another pet following a loss is an individual decision.
- It can depend on your life stage and the circumstances in which you find yourself.
- Being given a replacement pet without your consent may bring strong feelings of anger, as it interrupts the loss process. Sometimes it can be helpful, but it can also make a grieving owner feel unable to control the process of adapting to life without their former pet.
- Introducing a new pet into your home too early can lead to feeling that there is no closure on the previous pet, or to a feeling of disloyalty to the pet that has just passed away.
- Introducing a new pet after a former pet has gone missing can be particularly difficult.

The decision to share your life with another pet is one that only you can make. It will take time to move away from the grief following your previous loss. Take time to think about what you want.

Conclusion

Coping with any loss requires a period of psychological adjustment. We need time to accept the loss and to mourn. The process of mourning can be a healing one, but in experiencing the different reactions we can be faced with uncomfortable memories and raw emotions. The depth of our loss is shown both in the feelings we express and also in those we feel unable to show to others.

Losing a pet that has been a part of our life can make us feel that we have lost a part of our own history through shared experiences and memories. Our customs, beliefs and culture all play a part in how we create meaning from the role that our pets have played in our lives. Our hope must be that we can celebrate the life we have recently lost. Even when the circumstances have been such that we feel anger and rage, in time we will recover sufficiently to find calm again.

Pets are instinctively very resourceful. They find a way out of numerous problems by using their intuition and intelligence. They communicate both to each other and to us, and that communication strengthens the bonds that exist between them and us. The loss of a pet demands that we too are resourceful, and that we find ways to cope with the loss that we have experienced. Although not an easy task, it is one that can, in time, allow us to grow.

In death as in life, it is right that animals are entitled to ethical treatment, especially when facing the end of their lives. Those who have pets living with them would wish this to be the case, and hope that they themselves will be afforded the respect and dignity of having experienced a loss when their pets are no longer with them. Your own moving on can be helped by your wish for your pets to have a good ending and the knowledge that you were there to support them. This knowledge will help you to accept your loss.

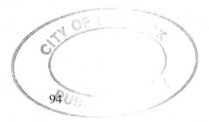

Useful addresses

Association of Pet Cemeteries
c/o Paws to Rest
Coombs View
Nunn Close
Armathwaite
Carlisle CA4 9TJ
Tel.: 016974 72232
The association has a code of practice and lists pet crematoria across
the UK.

Age Concern
Information Line
Freepost (SWB 30375)
Ashburton
Devon TQ13 7ZZ
Freephone 0800 00 99 66 (8 a.m. to 7 p.m. seven days a week)
Website: www.ageconcern.org.uk

Battersea Dogs and Cats Home
4 Battersea Park Road
London SW8 4AA
Tel.: 020 7622 3626
Lost and Found Line: 0901 477 8477 (within M25 area)
Website: www.dogshome.org
Email: info@dogshome.org

British Association for Counselling and Psychotherapy
BACP House
35–37 Albert Street
Rugby
Warwickshire CV21 2SG
Tel.: 0870 443 5252
Website: www.bacp.org.uk
Email: bacp@bacp.org.uk

British Psychological Society
St Andrew's House
48 Princess Road East
Leicester LE1 7DR
Tel.: 0116 254 9568
Website: www.bps.org.uk
Email: mail@bps.org.uk

Cambridge Pet Crematorium
A505 Main Road
Thriplow Heath
Royston
Hertfordshire SG8 7RR
Tel.: 01763 208295
Website: www.cpc-net.co.uk
Email: mail@cpc-net.co.uk

Council for Complementary and Alternative Medicine
179 Gloucester Place
London NW1 6DX
Tel.: 020 7724 9103

Cruse Bereavement Care
Cruse House
126 Sheen Road
Richmond
Surrey TW9 1UR
Helpline: 0870 167 1677
Website: www.crusebereavementcare.org.uk
Email: helpline@crusebereavementcare.org.uk

Cruse Bereavement Care Cymru
Ty Energlyn
Heol Las
Caerphilly CF83 2TT
Tel.: 029 2088 6913
Email: cruse.cymru@care4free.net

Cruse Bereavement Care Scotland
Riverview House
Friarton Road

Perth PH2 8DF
Tel.: 01738 444178
Website: crusescotland.org.uk
Email: info@crusescotland.org.uk

Northern Ireland Regional Office
Piney Ridge
Knockbracken Healthcare Park
Saintfield Road
Belfast BT8 8BH
Tel.: 028 90 792419
Email: annet@crusebereavementcare.org.uk

Doglost.co.uk is an internet-based dog registration scheme which helps reunite lost dogs with owners.
General enquiries: 01909 730077. If your dog is missing: 01909 733366.
Website: www.doglost.co.uk

Guide Dogs for the Blind Association
Burghfield Common
Reading
Berkshire RG7 3YG
Tel.: 0118 983 5555
Website: www.guidedogs.org.uk
Email: guidedogs@guidedogs.org.uk

Hearing Dogs for Deaf People
The Grange
Wycombe Road
Saunderton
Princes Risborough
Bucks HP27 9NS
Tel.: 01844 348100

The Beatrice Wright Training Centre
Hull Road
Cliffe
Selby
North Yorkshire
YO8 6NG
Tel.: 01757 638666

Website: www.hearing-dogs.co.uk
Email: info@hearing-dogs.co.uk

Help the Aged
207–211 Pentonville Road
London N1 9UZ
Tel.: 020 7278 1114
Website: helptheaged.org.uk
Email: info@helptheaged.org.uk
Send an A5 envelope to receive a free leaflet, *Bereavement*, and an information sheet, *Beating the Blues*, to the Information Resources Team. They can also advise on insurance, etc.

Institute for Complementary Medicine
PO Box 194
London SE16 7QZ
Tel.: 020 7237 5165
Website: www.i-c-m.org.uk
Email: info@i-c-m.org.uk

Mind (National Association for Mental Health)
15–19 Broadway
London E15 4BQ
Tel.: 020 8519 2122 (Office)
MindinfoLine: 0845 766 0163
Website: www.mind.org.uk
Email: contact@mind.org.uk
Contacts for local branches are in local telephone directories

The National Federation of Private Pet Crematoria
has a Directory of UK pet crematoria. Details are listed at:
www.petcrematoria.org.uk
Further national listings of pet cemeteries and crematoria can be found on 118.com; searches can be refined to regional areas.

NHS Direct
Tel.: 0845 4647
Website: www.nhsdirect.nhs.uk

People's Dispensary for Sick Animals (PDSA)
Head Office
Whitechapel Way
Priorslee
Telford
Shropshire TF2 9PQ
Tel.: 0800 917 2509
Website: www.pdsa.org.uk

Pet Bereavement Support Service
The Blue Cross
Shilton Road
Burford
Oxon OX18 4PF
Tel.: 01993 822651
Helpline: 0800 096 6606 (8.30 a.m. to 8.30 p.m. seven days a week)
Website: www.bluecross.org.uk
Email: pbss@bluecross.org.uk

Pet Travel Passports
c/o Department of Environment, Food and Rural Affairs (DEFRA)
Defra general helpline: 08459 33 55 77
Website: www.defra.gov.uk
(Other helpful websites: www.petplanet.co.uk; www.britishembassy.
gov.uk)
Email: helpline@defra.gsi.gov.uk

Pets as Therapy
PO Box 11
Stanley
Co. Durham DH9 7YZ
Tel.: 0800 917 2509
Website: www.petsastherapy.org

The Place2Be
Wapping Telephone Exchange
Royal Mint Street
London E1 8LQ
Tel.: 020 7780 6189
Website: www.theplace2be.org.uk
Email: enquiries@theplace2be.org.uk

Charity that offers emotional and therapeutic support to children in primary schools to help them deal with problems of all kinds.

Society for Companion Animal Studies
The Blue Cross
Shilton Road
Burford
Oxon OX18 4PF
Tel.: 01993 825597
Website: www.scas.org.uk
Email: info@scas.org.uk

United Kingdom Council for Psychotherapy
2nd Floor,
Edward House
2 Wakley Street
London EC1V 7LT
Tel.: 020 7014 9955
Email: info@psychotherapy.org.uk

Yoga
A UK directory of yoga courses and classes can be found at: www.yoga4health.biz

References

1 S. Barker (1999) 'Therapeutic Aspects of the Human-Companion Animal Interaction', *Psychiatric Times*, **XVI** (2).
2 W. P. Anderson et al. (1992) 'Pet Ownership and Risk Factors for Cardiovascular Disease', *Medical Journal of Australia*, **157** (5), pp. 298–301.
3 E. Kübler-Ross (1969) *On Death and Dying*, p. 3. London: Routledge.
4 D. Dembicki et al. (1996) 'Pet Ownership May Be a Factor in Improved Health of the Elderly', *Journal of Nutrition for the Elderly*, **15** (3), pp. 15–31.
5 J. Serpell (1991) 'Beneficial Effects of Pet Ownership on Some Aspects of Human Health and Behaviour', *Journal of the Royal Society of Medicine*, **84** (12), pp. 717–20.
6 D. Lago et al. (1989) 'Companion Animals, Attitudes Towards Pets and Health Outcomes Among the Elderly: a long term follow up', *Anthrozoös* **3**, pp. 25–34.
7 C. Ness (2001) *Secrets of Dreams*, pp. 156–7. London: Dorling Kindersley.
8 H. Neiburg and A. Fischer (1982) *Pet Loss: A Thoughtful Guide for Adults and Children*, p. 80. New York: HarperPerennial.

Further reading

Barton-Rodd, Cheri, and Baron-Sorensen, Jane, *Pet Loss and Human Emotion*. Bristol, PA: Accelerated Development, 1998.

Harris, Julia, *Pet Loss: A Spiritual Guide*. New York: Lantern Books, 2002.

Heegaard, Marge, *When Someone Has a Very Serious Illness: Children Can Cope with Loss and Change*. Chapmanville, WV: Woodland Press, 1991.

Ironside, Virginia, *Goodbye, Dear Friend*. London: Robson Books, 1996.

Kowalski, Gary, *Goodbye, Friend: Healing Wisdom for Anyone Who Has Ever Lost a Pet*. Enfield, Middlesex: Stillpoint Publishing/ Airlift Book Company, 1997.

Kübler-Ross, Elisabeth, *On Death and Dying*. London: Routledge, 1969.

Lee, Laura, and Lee, Martyn, *Absent Friend: Coping with the Loss of a Treasured Pet*. Lydney: Ringpress Books, 1992.

Murray Parkes, Colin, *Bereavement – Studies of Grief in Adult Life*. London: Penguin, 1972.

Morehead, Debby, *A Special Place for Charlee: A Child's Companion Through Pet Loss*. Broomfield, CO: Partners in Publishing, 1996.

Nieburg, Herbert A. and Fischer, Arlene, *Pet Loss: A Thoughtful Guide for Adults and Children*. New York: HarperPerennial, 1982.

Index

acceptance 38
adolescence 48–9
ambivalence 89
anger 31–4
anxiety 7, 30–1
ashes 38, 44
attachment 4, 5–7, 47–8

bargaining 29–30
Battersea Cats and Dogs Home 63
belief system 66
bond 7, 10, 78
Bowlby, John 5, 46
Buddhism 6
burial 44, 47

cats 19–20, 52–3, 58
ceremonies 44, 84–5
children 6, 42–59, 62
Christianity 6
counselling-psychotherapy 40–1, 60, 88
cremation 22–3
culture 23, 83

death 21–2, 42–3, 46–7
denial 27, 28, 46
depression 36–7, 39–40, 60
disbelief 28
dreams 83–4
dogs (*see also* Guide Dogs) 64, 72–3, 78–81
doubts 18–19

elders 25, 71–7
environment 49
euthanasia 14–21

farewell room 23
finance 72

goldfish 42
Greyfriars Bobby 85
grief, 37, 55–7, 66–70
Guide Dogs 78–80
guilt 34–6, 57, 64–5

health 8–9, 72
Hearing Dogs 80–1
hibernation 57
Hinduism 6
hope 66
horses 11–12

indecision 15
Islam 6

Kennel Club 63

language 51–2
learning disabilities 68–9
Levinson, Boris 5
life cycle 6, 42
Lincoln, Abraham 6
loss stages 26–39, 43–5, 50–3

memorials 57, 59, 85
memories 82–6
missing pets 57–8, 61–5
mourning (tasks of) 43–5

myths 24–6

pet theft 62–4
Pets as Therapy 76
photos 45, 60
ponies (*see* horses)
psychic beliefs 67

relatives (and friends) 76
religion 23, 83
replacing (a pet) 74, 87–93
residential care 75

RSPCA 63

searching 30, 84
separation 7

tears 38
tortoise 57–8
travel 57

vets 32

young adults 59–60

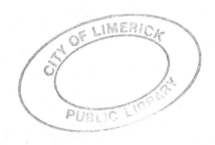